KT-552-199

# THE GOOD BACK GUIDE

# THE GOOD BACK GUIDE

BARRIE SAVORY D.O.

$$\overline{C}$$

Century · London

Published by Century in 2006

3 5 7 9 10 8 6 4

Copyright © Barrie Savory 2006

Barrie Savory has asserted his right under the Copyright, Designs and
Patents Act, 1988, to be identified as the author of this work

This book is sold subject to the condition that it shall not, by way of trade
or otherwise, be lent, resold, hired out, or otherwise circulated without
the publisher's prior consent in any form of binding or cover other than
that in which it is published and without a similar condition
including this condition being imposed on
the subsequent purchaser

First published in the United Kingdom in 2006 by Century
The Random House Group Limited
20 Vauxhall Bridge Road, London SW1V 2SA

Random House Australia (Py) Limited
20 Alfred Street, Milsons Point, Sydney,
New South Wales 2061, Australia

Random House New Zealand Limited
18 Poland Road, Glenfield, Auckland 10, New Zealand

Random House South Africa (Pty) Limited
Isle of Houghton, Corner of Boundary Road & Carse O'Gowrie,
Houghton 2198, South Africa

Random House Publishers India Private Limited
301 World Trade Tower, Hotel Intercontinental Grand Complex,
Barakhamba Lane, New Delhi 110 001, india

The Random House Group Limited Reg. No. 954009

www.randomhouse.co.uk

A CIP catalogue record for this book is available from the British Library
Papers used by Random House UK are natural, recyclable products
made from wood grown in sustainable forests. The manufacturing processes
conform to the environmental regulations of the country of origin

ISBN-13 9781844133965

Typeset by SX Composing DTP, Rayleigh, Essex
Printed and bound in Great Britain by
Antony Rowe Ltd, Chippenham, Wiltshire
Illustrations by Brian Robins

This book is concerned with non-specific back pain. The recommended
treatment is always given alongside, not instead of, other medical care. The
publisher and author expressly disclaim all liability to any secondary effects
of back trouble that may occur.

To Morland, Zena, Louise, Rosie, Martine, Alexander, Lauren, Michele, Maxine, Alastair and Melissa who are my past, present and future.

# ACKNOWLEDGEMENTS

To my secretary, Julia, for those extra bits of typing – she never complained.

To the team at Random House; Hannah Black for her editing, Ellie Clark for the publicity and to those behind the scenes for making it all happen.

To Brian Robins for managing to make proper illustrations frommy limited sketching ability.

To Alec Lom who introduced me to Century at Random House, and who pushed me along at the beginning.

To my wife, Rosie, who put up with my absences 'married' to the world processor.

And finally, to all my patients who have taught me so much.

# CONTENTS

# FOREWORD

I have spent many hours in the pilot's seat of a helicopter throughout my naval career and I have not been immune to the ergonomic failures of seating arrangements in aircraft.

We are generally considered to be increasingly sedentary in our society and the occurrences of musculo-skeletal problems are, as a result, becoming a major problem in our everyday lives.

The need to learn how to sit correctly and how to help ourselves recover from sitting with an incorrect posture is vital in countering musculo-skeletal problems, particularly as we now spend so much time in front of a computer screen.

Barrie's book so clearly illustrates these problems and imparts his knowledge and skills to allow each of us to help ourselves. Thus we can either prevent musculo-skeletal problems from ever occuring or remedy them by taking the correct actions to alleviate their consequences.

I have benefitted from Barrie's skill for many years and the knowledge, expertise and experience that he has built up from more than 40 years in practice will, I hope, bring much relief to many. It will help a wider audience understand that moving from tree to grassland has affected our skeletal structure and that with a little more care and attention we can learn to work with our body's design rather than against it.

HRH The Duke of York

# 1 IN THE BEGINNING . . .

Think of this as not so much an 'introduction', but more of a 'beginning'. This is a book about you and me, the human animal, and about the apparent paradox as to why, on the one hand, we are undoubtedly the most successful animals on the planet – even the universe – yet on the other, we are the only ones to suffer from epidemic levels of back pain. At first sight, the two can seem incompatible but, at a closer look, the first is really the cause of the second.

Since the middle of last century, our modern world has accelerated at an unprecedented pace and indeed shows no sign of slowing down. Our modern media has permitted the spread of ideas faster than at any other time in our history. The trouble is that this evolution of ideas has outstripped the evolution of our body's structure.

We are like the pigs in George Orwell's *Animal Farm* that eventually move in to Farmer Jones's farmhouse where they look totally out of place, trying to sit in the armchairs, eat at the kitchen table and sleep in the beds. Take away our clothes, and with it the very thin veneer of sophistication that we allow ourselves, then picture us sitting at our computer desks, driving our cars, slumping in our soft armchairs and squashing ourselves into plane seats. We look ridiculous. We quite simply don't fit into the world we have created. Let me give you an example.

## CURSE OF THE CURSOR!

CURSE stands for Continuous Use Repetitive Strain Effect. It applies to a myriad of situations, from the shoulder tension felt when driving on a motorway at night, to the muscular tension in the forearm from controlling the cursor on a computer screen with a mouse.

Take a moment to understand what happens when you use a mouse. The instant you hold the mouse you send a signal along a nerve from the brain – your body's central computer – to the muscles of your forearm and hand. It's like watching an old Wild West film where the 'baddies' light the fuse to a stick of dynamite. The flame zaps along it and eventually causes an explosion. Your thought ignites a chemical reaction along a nerve pathway until it reaches the intended muscle. The 'explosion' is an electrical discharge at the nerve/muscle junction, which causes the muscle to contract. This is a process that is going on consciously, and unconsciously, all day 24/7.

We're active animals, with our muscles instigating and controlling our movements, be it from turning our heads, picking up a cup or simply walking. But we're neither structurally nor functionally designed to hold muscles in contraction for long periods of time, just as we do when holding the muscles in the forearm tense to control the mouse.

Every contraction of a muscle requires energy; this energy comes in the form of a starch called glycogen in the blood supply. Arteries, with their muscular walls, pump blood into muscle tissue, energy is released to contract the muscle fibres, and lactic acid is produced as a residue.

Normally the movement of a muscle, a contraction and relaxation, helps as a pumping action on veins to drain lactic acid from the area (venous drainage). But if the muscle is consuming energy and producing lactic acid but remaining permanently contracted, then it's unable to produce the necessary pumping action for the efficient drainage of the veins. The result is that lactic acid builds up in the muscle fibres, rendering them hard and painful. Meanwhile the repetitive use of the same neural pathway 'burns' a permanent circuit in the system. The whole effect is a constant neural signal producing a contracted hardened muscle that is permanently bathed in lactic acid. It becomes impossible to consciously relax the muscle, resulting in pain and stiffness.

## THE REPETITIVE STRAIN EFFECT

The evolutionary idea that has produced the computer and the mouse has been far faster than the evolution of the structural and functional ability of the body to cope with it. It could be argued that we were better off when we used the old upright Imperial typewriter, where we had to make that sweeping movement, with

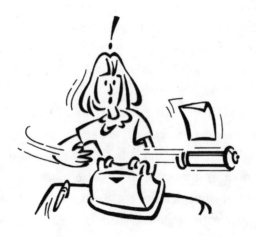

the right hand, to return the carriage to the start at the end of each line, and had to use a more exaggerated finger movement to depress the keys. Those movements, repeated every few seconds, were the necessary squeezing action of the forearm muscles to ensure the 'pumping' motion for the venous drainage. As one friend remarked, 'If only the Imperial had contained a cut and paste function, all would have been fine.'

## UPPER AND LOWER BACK
The majority of back problems, other than those caused by injuries of excessive force and strain, are due to the widening gap between the pace of the evolution of ideas and technology and the comparative slowness of the evolution of our bodies. These problems frequently blight our everyday lives.

While lower back problems are often the result of our difficulties in standing upright – and so working against gravity – with a lumbar spine increasingly weakened by our excessively sedentary lifestyle, problems with the upper back, neck and shoulders, are the result of our interfacing with the world of evolving ideas. A sedentary office life glued to the computer has become our biggest enemy.

## WHY SHOULD YOU READ THIS BOOK?
Recently receiving the practical details of how to collect my pension made me realise that I must now be cast in the role of elder statesman in my profession. It also made me realise that I have been promising to write this book for years and it is high time I got on with it. Forty years of treating, teaching and

learning from both patients and students has given me a unique insight into how we function, what goes wrong and, importantly, what can be done to correct it. I have always tried, and I hope succeeded, in explaining to patients in words, and examples that they can understand, the cause and the reason for their problems.

Having had one of the busiest practices in London, and over such a long time, has enabled me to knock around ideas with a broad spectrum of people. For many of my patients and friends the ideas expressed here are old hat. I have never been one to keep my light under a bushel. To those with whom I have not had the pleasure of one-to-one connection, I hope that this combination of a lifetime's work and ideas will be both useful and informative.

## STANDING UPRIGHT

Around 3.6 million years ago a simple event was captured for posterity, giving us a brief but tangible glimpse of the presence of our ancestors on this planet. Three sets of footprints were inexorably imprinted in wet volcanic ash freshly blown from the nearby Sadiman volcano in what is now modern Tanzania. One figure was in front, the second almost following directly behind and the third, slightly smaller, behind up and to the left.

These now famous Laetoli footprints show that they were hominids, human-like animals, and that they were standing upright. Were they a family with a child? Where were they going? How did they communicate? And, for the purpose of our statistics, did they have back pain, shoulder problems and headaches? Unfortunately, there are too few frames of even this quality for us to piece together a picture of our past.

Our nearest relative, the chimpanzee, can stand upright for periods of time, and so we can conclude, that evolving over millions of years, we must have gradually improved upon this attribute. In fact we haven't changed much physically – we share some 99 per cent of our genes with chimpanzees – but where we have changed is intellectually. Put in simple terms, that means if we had two bags of Lego, in the form of genes, one to build the human animal and the other a chimp, we could swap 99 pieces in every hundred and, in theory, still end up with our objective. But, in contrast to the chimps, for some reason we have been able to access our brain – our computer – to load and run an exceptional quantity, and quality, of 'software programmes'.

Geneticists suggest that women chose the more intelligent male as their partner, thus producing more intelligent offspring, and in this manner we have progressed to our current level of intellectual capacity. In a way, this intellect, and with it curiosity, came upon us a little too quickly and it has evolved at a seemingly unrestricted pace. We could have done with a few more million years, perfecting the change from walking on all fours to standing upright. This may well have resulted in a spine better adapted to sitting and standing in an upright manner than the one we currently have.

## SURVIVAL OF THE ECONOMICALLY FITTEST

I have a lovely 75-year-old gardener who looks after the land around our house in France. He has lived in a small hamlet, in a modest house, and looked after gardens and the land all his life. You can see just from looking at him that he is a happy man.

I said to him one day, 'Roger, never envy those who left the villages and went to the city to seek money and fortune. They all crave enough money to retire and do what you have done all your life!'

We settle for long hours in appalling conditions, facing the one-eyed monster of the computer, a slave to its presence. Though we earn more money, in real terms our disposable income, once we have paid the outrageous sums for just surviving in this expensive world of ours, leaves little left over.

The price we pay for this version of Utopia is a massive increase in back pain. Instead of the promised earlier retirement, and greater leisure, we are now facing the need to work even longer. Our increasingly sedentary existence weakens us further and, unless we learn how to adapt, this will only worsen.

## A BRIGHT NOTE OF OPTIMISM

If what you have read so far seems to be all doom and gloom, then let me help change that to something far more optimistic. Let me inject some element of hope, in a belief that we, the human animal, can learn by our errors and use the intelligence that we undoubtedly have to truly improve our future.

We have to take a radical look at the workplace. It is our interfacing with it that leads to most neck and back problems. We must teach our children how to avoid postural disasters as they slouch over the computer screen. We must devise a more 'user-friendly' environment. In the long run, the costs involved would be met by the savings in medical expenditure and the increased production of a workforce that is not weakened by back pain. We are at an unprecedented moment in our history and more than ever the future is potentially under our control. The baton has been passed to the next generation and they must improve on what we have done in the past.

Evolution is, and always has been, about survival. This book is about surviving, by understanding the problems we face in the modern world and, with that knowledge, being able to intelligently command our future. Back pain may not be fatal, but – as you'll know – it does affect the quality of our lives, and that's important. We have to learn to survive today, under today's circumstances, and it is to this end that I have written this book.

# 2 BACK PAIN: HOW DID WE GET INTO THIS STATE?

The human animal made two errors: the first was standing upright; the second was leaving our natural environment. We might have evolved to survive the first had we not rushed into the second.

When we embarked on a journey of scientific and intellectual evolution, we not only defined the moment of our success but also of our demise. Instead of evolving to live in harmony with our environment, we created the environment in which we live and have, ironically, become the victims of our own creation.

So while we have successfully become the most – or perhaps the only – intellectually developed animal on this planet, we are also the animal most poorly adapted to its environment. No longer are we in a world of survival of the fittest, but rather a world of survival of the economically fittest, and the economically fittest are, for the most part, urban-based and sedentary. And by driving our children to and from school, for example, we are teaching them to do the same.

Back pain is now filtering through to our teenage generation, as they sit uncomfortably at school desks, designed for yesterday's shorter generation, to return home to an evening sitting, slumped, in front of the TV or computer.

Unlike other animals, which have slowly and continuously adapted to their environment, we have bypassed that route. In previous generations we reached sexual maturity earlier, had many children and only the fittest survived – the planet's formula for progressive evolution.

Now, in our socially ordered society, we don't reproduce until later, have one or two children at the most, whom we can keep alive irrespective of the process of natural selection. In this state we can neither expect to have the time, nor turnover, to adapt to our environment. Natural selection would take far too long to produce the measures necessary for us to cope with our rapidly changing self-created world. The goalposts have moved, and are moving quickly, and our bodies simply can't keep pace with our minds.

It is no coincidence that over the last 50 years, there has been an unprecedented expansion in every sphere of intellect, but there has also been a catastrophic rise in the incidence of back pain. While our intellectual evolution, as shown by our material and scientific progress, rises at an astounding pace, the downside is that our physical demise matches it.

Current statistics from the Department of Health indicate that back pain is costing British industry some five billion pounds a year in lost production through absenteeism and the National Health Service (NHS) £481 million a year in treating it. The tragedy is that this is the UK's leading cause of disability, and even more disturbing is that recent research is showing that back pain is increasingly prevalent among children. These are NHS figures, and so do not include those who seek private help for their problems, or who suffer silently and struggle on with what they feel is an incurable situation. The real figure is probably much higher.

We are getting progressively weaker, less adapted, and thus less capable of coping with the world we have created. Our 'creature comforts' – the bed, the soft armchair, the car, the office desk and the computer – are the very instruments of our torture. Certainly, we are making some progress. We are now looking at user-friendly chairs, desks, and computers – and there is no doubt that these can help – but there is much more that we can and should be doing. We need a simple 'user-friendly guide' to the human animal, a straightforward, practical understanding of its structure, how it works and why it goes wrong. With this knowledge we can then find the logical solutions to cope with it.

Imagine that you have just opened the box of the latest new gizmo for your computer. You look at it with awe, admiration and a certain apprehension, and then look frantically into the almost discarded box, to search for that little plastic bag containing the 'Getting Started' and 'User's Guide' manuals. Well, this book is the 'Getting Started and User-Friendly Guide to the Human Animal'! So, sit back comfortably – a cushion in the small of your back, shoulders relaxed – and we can begin.

# 3 SETTING THE SCENE

One of the big problems about understanding ourselves is that we have become so familiar with our own shell and being that we simply take ourselves for granted. The old adage 'familiarity breeds contempt' is perhaps apt.

Take, for example, the fact that you are reading this book. You are using your three-dimensional, colour vision, binocular cameras. You are recording, comprehending, sifting and, hopefully, enjoying the experience. Yet hardly ever do we stop our hectic rush through life to take just a moment to be amazed at this, and all of the myriad miraculous processes that go to support our very existence.

For example, at the same time as you are reading this, you are busily pumping blood through your lungs, where it picks up oxygen in exchange for carbon dioxide, and then distributes it to every cell in your body. This is the very sustenance of your life. Your various organs and glands are automatically carrying out their allotted tasks in supporting your life.

You are a biomechanical miracle made up of muscles, bones, tendons, ligaments and fascia that are collectively called the musculo-skeletal system. An onboard computer, the brain, controls this system. Through the brain, and its network of wiring, the nervous system, lies the force that controls your entire functioning. Of all the collection of struts and levers in this machine that is you, there are none more miraculous and complicated than those that form the vertebral column or spine. It is no wonder that it is this structure, above all, that is the most vulnerable to injury and pain, especially as it is the spine that we humans use in such a different way to the rest of our vertebrate cousins.

We belong to a very large group of animals, the vertebrates, who share the common feature of possessing a vertebral column. Unfortunately, in some ways, we are the odd ones out. We are the only ones to use the vertebral column (spine) vertically. The rest of our close relatives remain essentially horizontal. That is one of our biggest problems.

Think of all the four-wheeled vehicles – buses, trains, lorries, cars – and imagine operating one of them vertically, balanced upright on the back wheels. Just imagine the engineering problems involved in making this happen – the modification to different systems, the stresses and strains placed on others.

Have you noticed how difficult it is to stand still? It's much easier to be on the move. Just like a cyclist trying to balance stationary, it's much easier to balance on the move. Later, I will explain the various problems brought about by our vertical posture, but for a moment I would like you to indulge in a little daydreaming.

## AN EXERCISE IN IMAGINATION

Abstract thought, which, in our daydreams and our little fantasies of imagination, we indulge in every day, is another of the unique gifts that we take for granted. Yet this facility, as far as we know, may be unique to the human animal.

We can imagine. We can imagine winning the Lottery and

what we might do with the winnings. We can imagine our planned summer holiday, with the sun, sea and sand.

So before we get down to the more serious matter of understanding how we work and why we go wrong, let's take a little trip in imagination. I would like you to 'step outside' yourself. Be the observer of you for a little while. Whoever is going on this trip is not your musculo-skeletal system, or even its back-up organs. It is not your brain, or any of the hardware that makes up your structure; it is something far less tangible. It is the unique you. Let's call it SELF.

So SELF come with me shopping. Let's really begin to make this a true SELF-help book. I want you to have the eyes of a child seeing something for the first time. We are going window-shopping. Your local computer store is doing a special promotion for its 'human machine' and, SELF, I would like you to have a look.

The store has agreed to a special viewing in its VIP suite so that you can see the full range of the product. The technicians are going to show you some examples of what it looks like and how it performs. So, SELF, just sit back in your chair and marvel at the experience.

First up on the screen is a clip from the first James Bond film, *Dr No*. Out from the sea steps the beautiful Ursula Andress, to be greeted by the young Sean Connery.

Next on screen is the famous performance by skating duo Torvill and Dean. Look at the balance, the grace, the control in their ice dance interpretation of Ravel's Bolero. We can then sneak a look at the great scientist Einstein stretching the limits of the human mind as he envisages the equation $E=MC^2$.

Perhaps to a little sport now? Maybe we can look at tennis ace Sampras winning Wimbledon, or the nail-biting Borg/McEnroe tie-break. Have a look for the moment at a clip of the Olympic gymnastic-winning performance of Nadia Comaneci. Marvel at her perfection of balance. The effortless grace perhaps of Olympic runner Sebastian Coe in full flight is worth a moment or two.

We could go on, but perhaps you have begun to see of what this human machine, this human animal, is capable. We have looked at the gems of human animal structure and function, spare now a moment to look at the rather sadder reality.

## A DAY IN THE LIFE OF . . .

SELF, this is what life can become. It's 6.30 a.m., you got to bed late having had dinner with friends. You drank too much. You have a headache and a hangover. Your back is playing up again after the gardening last weekend, and to crown it all you forgot to set the alarm earlier for your meeting at 7.30 this morning. You get out of bed bent over double, with your hands on the front of your thighs for support. Slowly, and somewhat painfully, you ease yourself into, almost, an upright position. You stagger inelegantly to the bathroom and look with horror at the vision that greets you from the mirror.

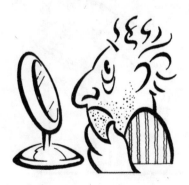

Washing is difficult as you are still unable to fully straighten your painful lower back.

You swallow, on an empty stomach, a couple of painkillers and make your way downstairs to grab a cup of instant coffee.

You are beginning to straighten up a little as you rush out to catch the train to get to the office in time. Stepping on to the train hurts your back again and it's painful to sit. You are just in time for the meeting but sitting for an hour is agony. The meeting over, the rest of the day is spent at your desk, hunched over the computer. You desperately try to find a comfortable way to sit and cope with your painful back. There's a panic at the office and lunch is a sandwich and coffee taken at your desk. You try to walk around and bend backwards to ease the pain, but sitting brings it back with a vengeance. The tops of your shoulders ache from the tension of sitting at the computer for so long, and to crown it all, you have a rotten headache under the base of the skull.

You look at the clock, it's 6 p.m. and you've promised you would go to a parents' meeting at the school. Do you face the wrath of your partner for missing the school appointment again, or, with so much work to get finished, the displeasure of your boss for leaving early?

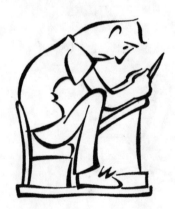

You leave work with a few hurried excuses to the boss, and a promise to finish the work at home later in the evening. Carrying a heavy briefcase, and a laptop, you dash to the station and push your way on to a crowded train. Nowhere to sit; so, painfully, you bend your 6ft 2in frame into a train designed for someone six inches shorter.

You race home, collect your partner and on to the school. Here you are sitting at a school desk designed for the under-tens. Embarrassingly, you twist and wriggle, trying to cope with the impossible. Bad-tempered, and in agony, you eventually get home where you then have to finish the report for tomorrow.

You finally slip into bed at 12.30, swallow another couple of painkillers, and lie awake trying to find a comfortable position for your wretched back, with tomorrow's report reverberating in your mind.

Well, it did seem fair to show you both sides of the coin. Let's assume that you have been more impressed by the upside than the down, and that, only for this week, the computer store is offering an amazing discount on a 'Full spec. human animal'. This comes with all the back-up systems, fully operational, just waiting for you to press the start button. Let's imagine that the machine you choose is in fact you. That's right, the very person sitting reading these words.

So the delivery guy has gone and left you with the cardboard container helpfully labelled 'this side up'. Excitedly you open the box, clear the bubble wrap and there you are in all your glory. Somewhat in awe, and with a certain trepidation, you look at this miracle of evolution, complete with all the working parts. All you have to do, as SELF, is to step inside and you are up and running. Hopefully, before you rush off into life, you stop for a moment with a sudden attack of panic. How do you operate it? How do you run it in? Do you run it in? How do you stop it? When do you stop it?

These are the questions you might have asked when you bought your first computer. So what do you do? You reach for the little plastic bag with the 'Getting Started' and 'User's Guide' manuals. In fact, SELF, abandon this off-the-shelf model and come with me now on a trip to the real world. We are going to get a new you. A unique, never-existed-before, you. This time, SELF, you can build it from scratch. Assemble it. Run it in. Enjoy it, expand it, try it to its limits, cruise in its middle years, and make the most of the latter ones.

# 4 GETTING STARTED: YOUR GUIDE TO THE BASICS

There are two pillars of wisdom that form the basis for understanding any living object, be it plant, bacterium, virus, or animal, and they are anatomy and physiology – in other words, structure and function. In order to better comprehend what we are, why we go wrong and, more importantly, what we can do about it, we do need to have some basic grounding in structure and function. Let's look at structure first.

## ASSEMBLING THE HUMAN ANIMAL

The reason why any anatomy textbook is so large is that every structure, be it internal organs or musculo-skeletal system, is described in minute detail. Fortunately, as we're only looking at our skeletal structures here, my aim, in the next few pages, is to give you a practical understanding of the complex mixture of struts and levers that together make up our musculo-skeletal system.

When everything is in working order, we take our bodies for granted, it's only when disorder – chaos – intervenes that we take notice. So in order to understand what goes wrong we need a simple understanding of how it all works and why symptoms occur when faults arise.

## THE MUSCULO-SKELETAL SYSTEM

A few weeks ago I watched an experienced operator delicately controlling one of those mechanical diggers. He sat in the cab, seemingly disconnected from the series of struts and levers that were engaged in lifting old tree roots from the garden, but in total control of the moving parts. Cut away the frills and fancies, and we are just a series of struts and levers, operated by a man in a cab. For us it's our arms and hands that make for such delicacy of control.

This was never more obvious to me than when I was asked to see a woman with an injury to her left elbow. She had sustained a fracture of her lower arm that included her elbow joint, and had become fixed in a permanently half-bent position so that she was quite unable to bring her left hand to her mouth. Try it for yourself – without bending the elbow it's virtually impossible to get your hand anywhere near your mouth. It just emphasises the intricacies of our structure, how we take for granted the apparently simple task of bringing a hand to the mouth.

If the mechanical digger was impressive, just look at what we can achieve with our series of struts and levers. Though we are made of lots of different-looking bones and joints that are built and perform in subtly different ways, realistically they are all much the same. So all that is necessary is to merely understand how one joint is built and works, then we can apply that knowledge to the rest. The easiest way to see how a structure is built is to build it.

The building-up of a Joint

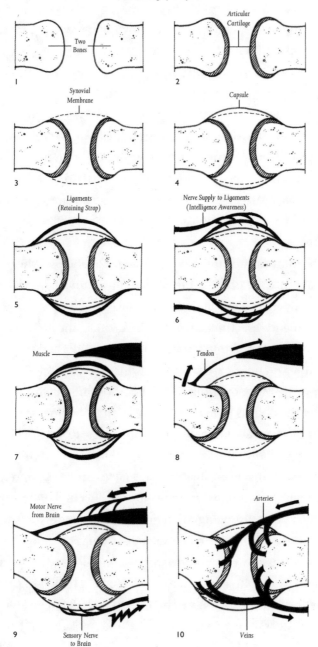

## Building a joint

1  A joint is the junction between two bones where movement can take place.

2  Articular cartilage is the silicon-like surface that allows one surface to glide smoothly over another. It's that glistening white surface that you see on the knuckle of a chicken leg. This is the bearing surface to stop the bone wearing away.

3  Synovial membrane is the inner lining of the joint that, as the joint moves, provides the special fluid that keeps the articular cartilage continually bathed in joint oil. Every movement of the joint 'milks' a continuous flow of synovial fluid.

4  The joint capsule is the outer casing that encloses the joint to make it a 'sealed for life' unit. The synovial membrane is effectively the lining of the capsule.

5  Ligaments are thickened bands, outside the joint capsule, that protect the joint from moving too far. They act like the leather retaining strap on the 'Mini' door. You are supposed to control the opening of the door, but if you should let go and the door is blown forcefully open by a wind, it takes the strain. A sprained ligament is when you tear or overstretch the ligament.

6  Ligaments have another very special function, beyond that of a retaining strap, in that they are intelligently aware of how much they are being stretched. This awareness is the very basis of how the musculo-skeletal system is held together and functions. Through a network of millions of tiny nerve endings sensitive to stretch, ligaments provide a constant feedback information mechanism of our spatial awareness.

7  Muscles are the active power units that make joints move.

8  Tendons are the 'ropes' that connect muscles to the bones.

9  Nerves are the cables that carry information to and from each joint. *Motor nerves* from the brain send signals to contract a muscle; *sensory nerves* carry information back to the brain on the position of the joint – where it is in space.

10  Blood vessels, arteries and veins, respectively, bring blood supply in and drainage out, providing energy, nutrition and health for the joint.

In ten simple steps, that's all you need to know for a basic understanding of what a joint is and how is it built. After that the musculo-skeletal system is just what it says – that system of bones, muscles and the stuff that joins them together to form the skeleton. Anything that goes wrong with this system is called a musculo-skeletal problem. So is, in fact, musculo-skeletal pain.

Fascia facts

Fascia, like ligament, is connective tissue. This means it connects things together. In fact, fascia connects the whole body together. Have you ever had a deep cut that goes down to a white layer under the skin? Well, that was fascia.

Though you may not know much about it, you have more fascia in your body than any other substance. It's like a type of protective clingfilm, enveloping every structure in the body – over bone, under skin, surrounding muscles, and organs (heart, lungs, kidneys, etc.). It is the same stuff you peel off from a kidney or heart, or the white sheet along a piece of meat.

Imagine you could immerse a body in a bath of special acid and select to dissolve everything except fascia. You would be left with a rather messy mass of white tripe. Now if you could blow it up, rather like blowing up one of those large lilos, you would gradually find that you had a sort of Michelin Man lilo, a complete human shape. Just a human lilo with all the shapes of organs inside but without the structure of bone, muscles and organs.

Now realise that, just like ligaments, fascia is full of nerve endings that again send up messages to the central 'computer' informing it of where you are in space.

## THE VERTEBRAL COLUMN

Each bone in the spine is called a vertebra and, together, they make up the vertebral column.

The vertebral column is divided into different regions:

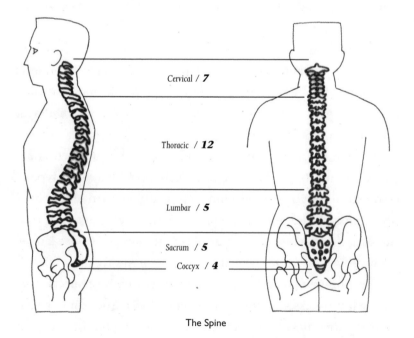

Cervical / **7**

Thoracic / **12**

Lumbar / **5**

Sacrum / **5**

Coccyx / **4**

The Spine

| The neck or cervical spine | 7 vertebrae. |
| The dorsal or thoracic spine | 12 vertebrae. |
| The lumbar spine or lower back | 5 vertebrae. |

These are the mobile segments, and then there are the fused (non-mobile) elements – the sacrum and the coccyx:

The sacrum, the triangular-shaped bone at the base of the spine, is made of five vertebrae fused together.

The coccyx, our tailbone remnant, consists of four bones fused together.

Each mobile vertebra is separated, and joined to the next, by a disc. Think of a disc as being like a car tyre, but blown up with fluid, not air. The biggest problem with a disc, judging by the number of faults that occur, is that it seems to be the structure that has least adapted to our upright posture. The rest of our vertebrate relatives, rather more sensibly, have remained essentially horizontal and do not insult the disc by constantly loading it vertically.

Any engineering manufacturer, on finding that a component part was frequently breaking down, would attempt to develop this structure further in order to improve the product. A car manufacturer would have long ago recalled this model to replace the faulty unit! Unlike car tyres, however, you cannot blow up a vertebra again if it bursts.

Though we belong to that group of animals called vertebrates, sharing the common feature of a vertebral column, our uncommon feature is that we chose to stand upright, and use the spine in a vertical position, a decision that has led to our back pain disasters.

Just one more piece of anatomy and I promise that's it. This concerns the part where the spine meets the legs, where the legs come up to the pelvis and the spine meets the pelvis. The base of the spine is called the sacrum and the bit of pelvis that meets the sacrum is called the iliac bone. The joint is the sacroiliac

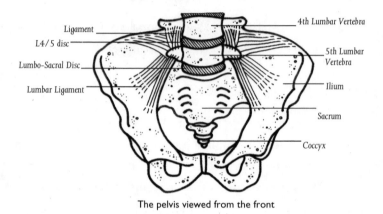

The pelvis viewed from the front

joint. It is like a keystone in an arch. It has become, in our upright posture, the single most load-bearing unit in the body. The trouble is it was meant to be a non-weight-bearing structure.

It's where we made the monumental change, from horizontal animal to vertical one, by going through 90 degrees at the hip joint and thus turning the sacroiliac joint from a horizontal, non-weight-bearing structure, to the most weight-bearing structure in the body. No wonder back pain is so common.

## THE OPERATING SYSTEM

Now that we've looked at structure it's time to move on to function and to look at two words, and their concepts, that are

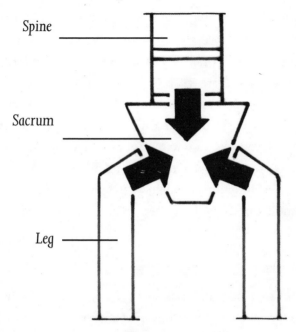

Spine

Sacrum

Leg

**Sacrum as the keystone of an arch**
*Three forces of the body pass through the sacrum*

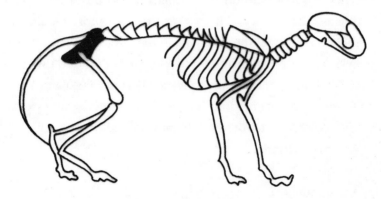

**Four-legged animals have a horizontal sacrum which
is not weight-bearing**

the key to understanding how our structures work. These are 'posture' and 'proprioception'

I'm sure that everyone is familiar with the word 'posture'. But I would wager that there will be few people who have heard of the word 'proprioception', and certainly fewer who could describe it. Yet, just as our whole lives are involved in some way or another with posture, so every moment of our existence has some aspect of proprioception. Between 'posture' and 'proprioception' lies not only the very function of our bodies but also the faults. Some understanding of them both is essential.

POSTURE

Posture is very personal; it's almost as recognisable as a signature, or a fingerprint. My own definition of posture is, 'the individual's way of balancing their body in an upright position against the force of gravity'. We all do it in one way or another and we all vary slightly. Unfortunately some of our posture habits are potentially more harmful than others; in fact posture – whether sitting or standing – is at the very root of most of our back problems. We can't help having some sort of posture, as it's merely our act of balancing on two legs; what we don't want are excessive curves in the spine that then become a problem.

There are really only four basic types of standing posture, and we all fall into 'variations on a theme' around them.
- Kypho-lordotic.
- Sway back.
- Too straight.
- Scoliosis.

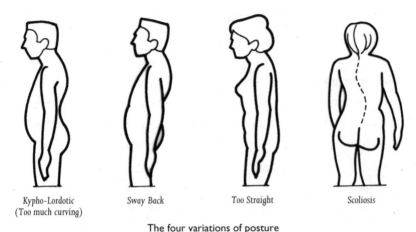

Kypho-Lordotic          Sway Back          Too Straight          Scoliosis
(Too much curving)

The four variations of posture

### Kypho-lordotic

'Kyphos' describes a bowing outwards of the spinal curve, as in the thoracic spine, and 'lordosis' is the bowing inwards. One could also use the terms 'concave' and 'convex', or 'flexion' and 'extension', as they all essentially describe the same shape.

We all need some degree of bending, flexion and extension in our spines to give it an element of flexibility, so that it can act like the leaf springs on a car chassis that allow for bounce and shock absorption. Kypho-lordosis really applies to an excessive curve that then becomes a postural problem.

### Sway back

This is where the pelvis and tops of the thighs move forwards and the upper body leans backwards, to provide a counterbalance. If one were to draw in an imaginary line of gravity, it would fall behind the base of the spine. This is not a good posture in any form but particularly when standing, as the constant force trying to make you lean backwards leads to ligamentous back pain –

back pain associated with a problem with the ligaments (see page 99).

## Too straight

This is perhaps the least common posture, but nevertheless significant, in that a too-straight spine prevents the shock-absorbing function that some gentle curves would offer.

## Scoliosis

Scoliosis is the odd one out as this is a lateral curve, where the others all refer to a 'fore and aft' balance, and this can exist in conjunction with the other three.

Lateral curves may be purely temporary, as with an acute muscle spasm asymmetrically pulling you over to one side, or as a more permanent problem due to a fault in the development of the spine during the years of teenage growth.

With the presentation of an acute scoliosis, though it may look alarming, it is self-limiting and the spine returns to normal when the muscle spasm resolves.

A developmental scoliosis may be potentially more serious as once the lateral 'S' shape goes beyond a critical angle, then the body weight will further accentuate the curve and may lead to a dangerous situation that will require a surgical solution. It is essential to note lateral curves early in a child's development as with the right treatment they can be controlled and in the majority of instances surgery prevented.

Our sitting postures, for such large parts of our lives, have become our disaster scenarios.

## PROPRIOCEPTION

The key to understanding our whole musculo-skeletal system, and as to how it works, is to be aware of how the connective tissues (fascia and ligaments) integrate with the muscles to make us function.

Nerve endings fire back information from the stretch and pressure receptors in the muscles of the connective tissue (fascia and ligament), to give you an awareness of where you are in space. I love the description once made by the wonderful sports commentator Ron Pickering. He not only had a superb understanding of his subject, but he also brought a wonderful sense of infectious enthusiasm to his commentaries. On this occasion, he was commentating at the Olympic Gymnastics, when watching a complicated, faultless vault by Nadia Comaneci, involving somersaults and twists, when he said, 'Oh my goodness, what an incredible sense of spatial awareness.' His technical appreciation of exactly what that vault required is not only a perfect example of spatial awareness, but it embraces the very essence of proprioception. I would like you to get a sense of this for yourself.

Let's imagine, for example, that you are reading this book sitting in a chair. I want you to focus your attention on your hands and fingers holding the book. Can you feel them? Now focus on the position of your elbows. Try to become aware of them. Next, feel the weight of your body on your backside and feel your spine against the back of the chair. If you are sitting with your legs crossed, feel the position of one on the other. Have a trip around and 'feel' all of you.

Subconsciously, all the time, every millimetre of you is sending information from your musculo-skeletal system to your brain. In consciously thinking of it, you brought it to your awareness, but this process was going on anyway. Even though you are now not focusing on those bits, they are still sending information.

About 100 years ago, the English neurologist Sherrington described it as 'the continual flow of sensory information from the periphery to the central cortex (brain)'. He called it 'proprioception'.

'Proprio' really means property. It's your perception, or feeling, of your property – in other words, you! If you can carry this idea of proprioception and your newly acquired knowledge of the musculo-skeletal system into the rest of the book, then you will have a greater understanding of all the things that can go wrong with your body and how to cope with them.

Everything we do, using our musculo-skeletal system, involves proprioception. It is the means by which our whole function is organised. From walking to writing, chewing to chatting, there is nothing that we can actively do that does not involve proprioception.

Probably one of the best examples is walking. Imagine you have a software programme in your 'computer' called 'WALK'. Whenever you wish to engage it, all you have to do is switch to 'walk mode' and it happens. You can get up from the chair you are in and walk to the kitchen and make a cup of tea. You do not even have to think about how to walk; it just happens.

Proprioceptive nerve endings in the sole of your foot, in the ligaments of your ankle, in the Achilles tendon of your heel, in your knee, hip, spine and neck all integrate to feed into your computer's sensory information from the periphery to the central computer. The 'software' that you long ago established, through conditioned reflex, runs 'walk mode' and sequentially orders exactly the right muscles, at the right time, to enable you to walk smoothly. This is all down to proprioception.

I have a favourite question that I love to ask when I am teaching a post-graduate class. 'Why do you limp when you sprain your ankle?' Usually the first reply is, 'because it hurts'. Of course that's true, as pain is one of the sensations transmitted by your sensory nerves from the damaged ligament fibres, but pain is not really the reason why you limp. You often still limp when the pain has gone. The explanation is this. We are a series of integrated circuits. When you walk, the series of nerve impulses from the different ligaments in your leg, particularly the foot and ankle, fire up to the central computer, which then sends a nerve impulse to the appropriate muscle telling it to contract. The whole integrated series of circuits allows for the smooth walk mode.

Now imagine that you damage a ligament in your ankle. The nerve endings from that section of ligament can no longer smoothly fire off information to the computer, for it to send a signal to the next muscle group. You have broken the circuit, so you miss a beat and limp. Limping, in that sense, is caused by the failure of your system to command the normal sequence of muscular contractions that is walk mode. With great effort you can try to override the involuntary limp, but lose attention for a moment and the limp will come back.

Understanding that feedback loop, and its application to our own body's systems, is the key to understanding most of the rest of this book. One way or another, all of our musculo-skeletal dysfunctions, be they low back pain or shoulder dysfunction, come back to a breakdown in some aspect of our biological feedback loops. Embracing that concept makes the rest easy. Now you can smoothly walk to the kitchen and make that cup of tea.

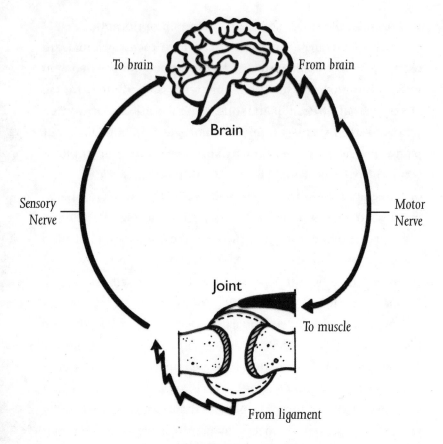

To brain            From brain

**Brain**

Sensory                        Motor
Nerve                          Nerve

**Joint**

To muscle

From ligament

**Feedback loop**

## THE SPINE: HOW IT WORKS AND WHAT CAN GO WRONG

Now for a closer look at the most complicated piece of the
musculo-skeletal system, the vertebral column. We have already
looked at its structure; now we need to understand its function.
As with any piece of machinery the more complicated it is, the
more likely is it to go wrong. This piece of our machinery is no
exception to that rule, as problems with the spine can dominate
our lives.

We may well go through life suffering little from pain in the shoulders, hips, elbows and knees, but it is a rare human animal that does not, at some time, suffer back pain. For some it is an ongoing persistent problem that dominates their whole existence; for others it creeps up on them without warning. For many, the medical phrase 'recurrent episodic back pain' is the apt description. For certain, if you've had it once, you are more likely to have it again.

In order to understand how and what goes wrong we have to delve a little into how the spine is built and how it works. Once you grasp this you need never again be at a loss to understand your own problems and may even be able to prevent a few more from occurring.

## Mutation miracle

Somewhere along our evolutionary past, a series of chance events, over millions of years, resulted in the vertebral column. It enabled animals to have a front end, and a back end, which could work independently of each other, joined by a flexi rod linking them together. The vertebral canal is a hollow core that houses the vital cables of the spinal cord. It forms a conduit that protects the vital nerves carrying information to and from the brain, the body's organising computer or control centre.

Having, in evolutionary terms, 'chanced' upon the building of a spine, it was as if nature then went on a frenzy of experiment. With a flexible, bony canal there was virtually no limit to the distance from the back legs to the front ones. We, the human animal – the cocky new kid on the block – are the only vertebrates to use the spine vertically and there lies the problem. To understand why standing upright is a problem we need to look at how the spine works horizontally and, in particular, to understand the functions of inter-vertebral discs, the spine and the pelvis.

### The discs

These are the comparatively soft units separating one vertebra from the next. It is they that give the flexibility to the spine. Remember, they are like car tyres blown up with fluid instead of air. The hard outer wall of the tyre is called the annulus, and the softer, pulpy core is called the nucleus pulposus. You can forget these two names; instead just think of the tyre wall and the thick pulpy fluid core. So now join 24 or so vertebrae and stick a disc between each one and you have the wonderful flexi rod of the spine.

### The pelvis

The pelvis is essentially a bony circle joining the two legs to the spine. It also houses and protects the whole of the reproductive kit and provides space for a couple of exhaust pipes, one for fluid and one for solid. The convenient bulky buttocks afford a suitable structure to sit on.

### The sacrum

This simple triangle of bone is one of the most important structures of the musculo-skeletal system. It is so special that the very name, derived from Greek, is from our word 'sacred'. In some ancient cultures it was thought to be the seat of the soul, or, in Indian spiritual philosophy, the point where *Kundilini*, the snake-like form, rises from the base of the spine to awaken the dormant spiritual core. Certainly, be it philosophical or physical, it is a unit of profound importance.

The sacrum is in fact made of up five bones/vertebrae fused together into one. Understanding how it works in all horizontal vertebrates allows us to see why it is the single biggest problem when we started to stand fully upright.

When you look at any animal standing on four legs, it is easy to see that the pelvis is narrower above and broader below. Also the angle of the sacral surfaces in contact with the rest of the pelvis at the ilia – hence sacroiliac joints – allows the sacrum to hang between the two sides. The sacrum 'floats' between the ilia, attached by the powerful sacroiliac ligaments. At the tail end is the tail. At the head end is the head. The two are joined by the flexi rod, the spine. The sacrum is a non-weight-bearing unit hanging between the sides of the pelvis.

In the horizontal position, the spine is a non-weight-bearing unit hanging between the front and back legs. The flexibility of this arrangement is magnificent. We see evidence of this in the way animals move.

I love watching those dog trials where the dogs have to twist between a series of upright poles. The way in which the dogs wriggle their spines, with obvious joy, always makes me marvel at their flexibility. See, too, how any of the cat family, from domestic kitten to sleek leopard, twist and turn in play and survival.

This miracle of evolutionary creation, the vertebral column, has been enjoyed by countless species, many now extinct, over several hundred millions of years. The precision engineering of each segment, with such flexible motion and yet such protection of the vital trunk of nerves, would be the envy of any design engineer today.

If you were to tell that engineer you have decided to make a radical change and run the machine vertically, he would throw his arms in the air in utter disbelief and despair. It's impossible! Yet us humans, this new twig on a branch of the tree of evolution, have done exactly that. But at a price!

## CORE MUSCLE STRENGTH AND THE ERECTOR SPINAE

'Core muscle strength', is very much the 'in' phrase, when talking about back pain prevention and treatment. As with so many things, I am sure that, for most, the words are bandied about with very little actual understanding of the structures and concepts involved.

There are five distinct layers of muscle that organise, move and balance the spine.

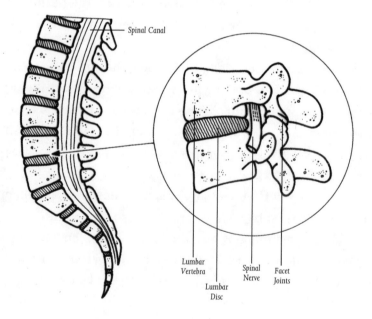

Lumbar Spine

If we start with the deepest layer first, which is the 'core' of the spine's control mechanism, we can build up our understanding of the rest.

The deepest layer of muscle, called the 'multifidus' and 'rotatores', is particularly specialised in its action and is essentially proprioceptive in function. Let me explain that last sentence, before a rather glazed look creeps into your eyes.

### The magician's magic wand

Sometime in the past, most of us have seen a magician do that trick of letting the magic wand bend in several places, and then miraculously restore it to a straight, rigid structure. All he did was to pull tight a string that runs up in the hollow of the wand, and restore it to its pristine state. Well, that's what the deepest layer of erector spinae muscles do to the spine. The only difference is that these muscles are not inside the hollow core of the spine but lie on the outer casing.

This deepest layer only runs from one vertebra to the next and serves to keep the spinal 'magic wand' straight, so that our 32 segments don't flop around. These muscles respond to nerve signals from the ligaments, which join each segment in the classic proprioceptive manner. Like any muscle group in the body, their tone – the resting state of readiness for action – is dependent on being trained by regular use. A muscle that is out of action for any appreciable period of time, and that can be measured in hours and days, not just weeks and months, loses its fine tune and becomes weaker. Anyone who has had an injury to a joint, such as the knee, will know how quickly that happens and how long – and how much effort – it takes to get that tone back.

This deepest layer is no exception and is particularly

vulnerable to lack of use. That's where sitting becomes such a problem. A sedentary lifestyle will rapidly lead to the loss of tone of our deepest layer of the erector spinae. Hours of slumping at the office desk and on the sofa in front of the TV take weeks of dedicated exercise to re-establish that tone again. Very few people would be prepared to dedicate the time and effort needed to achieve the change, so the moral is don't lose it in the first place.

The next layer of muscles spans three vertebrae, the next four vertebrae, and so on, until the most superficial layer spans six vertebrae. In essence, the deepest layer 'holds' the spine together while the outer layers instigate and control the movements that we use in our everyday lives. The big problem is that the more sedentary we have become, the more we have lost the natural background of muscle tone necessary for our spinal integrity. 'Use it or lose it' is the message.

### The performing seal

In order to visualise the spine's action, imagine a performing seal at a circus balancing on a round table with a ball on its nose. The seal wriggles underneath the ball, moving forwards and back, sideways and a bit of rotation, in an attempt to keep upright with the ball on its nose. This what our spine does in balancing the head on the neck.

Now, to rapturous applause, the seal flicks the ball to the trainer and with, an 'oink' 'oink', is rewarded with a couple of herrings. Seal and trainer exit stage left and now the spotlight dramatically focuses on the next act.

### The performing seal on stilts

The audience rises to its feet with unanimous cries of 'bravo, bravo' as on walks the performing seal on stilts, still balancing a ball on its nose.

Yes folks, that's us. The performing seal on stilts. That we manage this act at all is exceptional, that we do it with surprising ease does not take away from it the degree of difficulty involved.

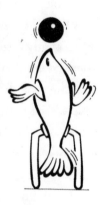

The cost, in engineering terms, of using structures vertically rather than horizontally, and the difficulty in balancing vertically, is enormous. The energy cost in balancing the spine vertically against gravity is a constant daily outgoing, in marked contrast to the far less demanding balancing on four legs. The weight-bearing load on ankles, knees, hips, sacrum and discs, that comes from standing on two legs instead of four, is the reason why these structures suffer so much from degenerative wear and tear, swelling the queues for joint replacement surgery.

This damage includes the gradual, and sometimes sudden,

squashing of the discs to produce a flat tyre with all its consequences. But perhaps the biggest change of all is to the small triangular bone, the sacrum. As we've seen, the sacrum is the keystone that fits between the two sides of the pelvis and it is here that we made the biggest change in standing upright.

We took a structure that, in four-legged horizontal vertebrates, is a non-weight-bearing hanging unit and made it into the most weight-bearing unit in the human animal. By turning 90 degrees at the hip joints and tilting the pelvis vertically, we changed everything. Now the pelvis is broader above and narrower below and the sacrum fits in between the two sides like the keystone of an arch. This keystone carries the whole weight of the spine and body above and the upward force of the legs from below. Not only does it support those loads, but it has to proprioceptively balance as well. Our performing seal meets the stilts at the sacroiliac joints. The ligaments of the sacroiliac joints have to 'propriocept' the spine above and the two legs below. This would not be too bad if we did not habitually stand on one leg.

### The drawer sideways in its runners

Just as balancing on a bicycle is easier when moving than when you are attempting to balance stationary, so we are better on the move than standing still. When standing still we hardly ever carry weight evenly on both legs. Take a look at any group of people standing, or rather slouching, and you'll see them leaning against a wall or continually shifting from one leg to the other.

We are very uncomfortable standing still and habitually carry our weight on one leg more than another. As we do so we put an uneven load on the sacrum that ends up like a drawer sideways in its runners, unable to move freely. So, instead of the sacrum being a free unit, distributing and balancing the three forces – two legs and the spine – it becomes the source of most of our lower back problems. But we will come back to that later.

### The balancing act

Let's go back to our performing seal and its balancing act. Balancing is a proprioceptive circuit. This means at any joint (a junction between two bones) there is a circuit between the ligaments supporting it and the muscles controlling it. The circuit is completed by nerves running from the ligaments to the brain and returning back again to the muscles controlling it.

Imagine you are trying to balance on one leg (try it tonight when you are cleaning your teeth). The ankle wobbles about a bit as the ligaments around the ankle fire up information to your brain that responds by contracting, or relaxing the right muscles to balance you.

Ballet dancers, who frequently sprain (or partially tear) ligaments, do a remedial exercise by standing on one leg on a breadboard over a tennis ball. This is, rather justifiably, called a wobble board! They are able to retrain the damaged neural circuits, the pathways of ligamentous proprioception, and re-establish a superb circuit, to the brain and back again. The better the circuit, the less likely they are to sprain the ankle again.

### The spinal wobble board

The spine is really a series of 'wobble boards' that we skilfully balance on each other against gravity. In this case, the successive boards sandwich 'the ball' between themselves. Fortunately, rather than using a ball, our discs spread the load evenly from one vertebra to the next, and the fluid core acts as a perfect hydraulic interface that transfers the weight smoothly.

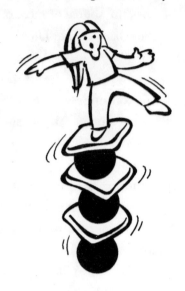

### Programming the body's computer

When we learnt to walk, very tentatively at first, we gradually loaded a software programme on to our computer's hard disc. Those first few steps, at about one year old, set the pattern of upright posture that distinguishes the human animal from its four-legged cousins. Our spinal wobble board, with one vertebra positioned on another and a disc in between, enables us to bend forwards, sideways and rotate, transferring the weight smoothly and evenly. So far so good.

We established this programme well and we use it every day without thinking about it. We get up from sitting, lying, get in and out of cars and walk almost without having to think.

Now let's throw a spanner in the works! *You have performed an illegal operation and will be shut down.* Those dreaded, insulting words from our computer's software, that seemingly arrive for no comprehensible reason, suddenly take on a different meaning.

Imagine we are cruising along nicely, running our performing seal without thinking. The combination of flexion, extension, side-bending and rotation accommodate all the movements we need. We take it for granted that it all works so well.

Now imagine that one of our discs, or tyres, has developed a flat – perhaps slowly, like a car left in the garage for six months, or maybe more acutely and suddenly. You cannot see it, you may not feel it, or be aware of it in any conscious way, but one of your tyres has lost its pressure and is about to give you a nasty shock. Tyre manufacturers are very particular about maintaining the right pressures to protect the tyre wall as a flat tyre will shear laterally when going round a bend.

So you have taken for granted your proprioceptive control of one vertebra connecting to the next via a disc. Now you, slightly too casually, reach down to pick up a pencil on the floor and wham! The flat tyre enables one vertebra to very slightly shear across the one below. You have no brain reference for this shearing motion, only for flexion, extension, side-bending and rotation. The unknown proprioceptive signals flash up to the software programme written on the hard disc in your body's computer centre and illuminate the screen with the message: *You have performed an illegal operation and will be shut down!* Your body's computer panics and immediately shuts down.

Order becomes chaos, as all the muscles relating to that unit go into an emergency, protective spasm, response. It is as if the 'foreign' signal triggers a confused response, resulting in overreaction. Your subconscious protection mechanisms sense that if the shearing motion is left unchecked, then you may shear in half, so the spasm locks you into position and, to put it mildly, you are stuffed. To get an idea of the power of this reaction, think how if you clench your jaw it is very difficult to forcefully open it against your will. The muscles at the base of the spine have supported your whole body weight for years and when they lock they are extremely powerful, as anyone suffering this problem will attest. This awareness of the body's protection mechanisms is the key to understanding most of our back problems. The rest are merely variations on this theme.

### Triangle between three forces

It is not unreasonable that the two structures which changed most when we began standing on two legs, the sacrum and the spine, should be the cause of most of our back problems. The sacrum, the arrowhead base of our performing seal, works pretty well until it gets wedged asymmetrically, like a drawer in a desk sideways in its runners, so that it cannot function properly. Let me show you what I mean.

Let's say you are standing balanced on your right leg. Your body weight is more loaded on the right side of the sacrum and the sacrum slides down and jams like the drawer.

When you stand it is easy to see, with a trained eye, the tilt of the pelvis so that the top of the sacrum, the base of the upturned triangle is on a slant. So our performing seal has to balance this sideways tilt before it does anything else. Instead of being able to use the muscles in the spine to balance vertically, you have to dedicate a large proportion of these muscles to stop yourself from falling sideways!

In addition, if you have a 'flat tyre', you have an unstable 'wobble board' on which to balance, and therefore must continually muscularly control that unit, in order not to throw the whole works out of order. Trying to balance the whole column of the spine on the titled triangular base and the even more unstable wobble board of the flat tyre disc, and you have a problem. Without realising it the muscles keeping the spine upright – the erector spinae – are working overtime just to stay in control. They are in a constant state of overactivity. In this condition they are vulnerable to further injury either by a sudden accident or from a continued exercise with which they lack the resilience to cope.

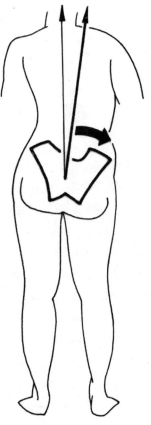

Standing on right leg

## THE BULGING DISC

Imagine the flat tyre. It may be just a slight pushing out of the wall, a barely perceptible bulge, or a more serious weakness leading to a herniation. The trouble is that structurally there's not much spare room before this bulge presses on a nerve root emerging from the spinal cord. Pressure on a nerve hurts.

Each nerve is made up of bundles of tiny fibres. Think of a

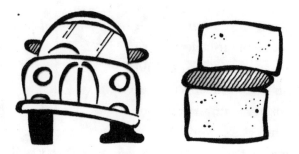

telephone engineer on a pavement pulling on a bunch of coloured wires that are disappearing into the ground. Information is going in and information is coming out. This is a nerve, a collection of lots of different wires, some sending information out and some sending it in.

The wires of the nerves going out are carrying commands such as to contract a muscle, while those coming in are carrying sensations such as pain or spatial awareness.

As with the telephone engineer, with his bunch of colour-coded wires, some may go to the house next door, others may be

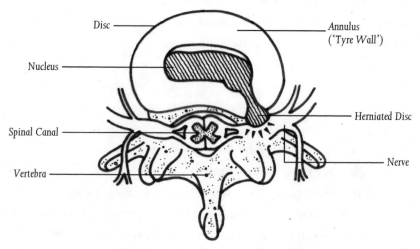

Bulging disc pressing on a nerve root

travelling a long way along the road. So, in a nerve, some of the fibres may go from the base of the spine to the big toe, others may just go to the side of the thigh.

The amount of pressure will determine the degree of interference produced and thus be reflected in the presenting symptoms that occur. Just a light touch on the cable and maybe all you will feel is a little tingling sensation a bit like pins and needles. Press  harder and the sense-feeling nerve – the sensory nerve – starts to lose its ability to feel. This may result in numbness or the loss of sensation.

With this level of pressure you will probably get some interference with the outgoing control nerves – motor nerves. This will cause a sort of choking of the nerve power and not enough nerve impulse to send signals along the cable to the muscles. The result is a loss of muscle power. It might mean that you couldn't stand on tiptoe on your left foot, or grip with your thumb and first finger, depending on the nerve involved. All of these can be tested by someone examining your reflexes.

There are probably few of us who have not had at some time the tap on the knee with a patella hammer to make the knee jerk. If the knee doesn't jerk when you tap the tendon below it, thus giving a sudden stretch to the proprioceptive receptors, then it probably indicates that pressure on a part of the nerve has been sufficient to break the circuit. At this stage there is almost certainly pain and a lot of it!

If you have ever had toothache, maybe due to pressure on a nerve from an abscess, then you know what nerve pain feels like. The nerve involved in a tooth is the thickness of a human hair, the nerve that runs down the back of the leg from the base of the spine, the sciatic nerve, is in comparison like a ballpoint pen refill. So it's hardly surprising that this really hurts! The pain is probably due to two things, direct pressure and inflammation.

## INFLAMMATION

When I was first studying my profession I could never really take in the idea of inflammation. For me inflammation was a septic process, like a pimple or a boil. I couldn't understand that in fact it is, very simply, the body's response to injury, and an integral part of its healing mechanism. Once I could see that, it made a big difference to my understanding of body function. Assuming that some of you may be a bit like me, let me give you an example that visually, and usually painfully, presents the various aspects of inflammation.

Let's say you buy a pair of shoes. They look great and you put them on to go to a wedding. Halfway through the church service they start to hurt. Thankfully you move on to a sit-down lunch and under the cover of the table you are able to ease them off your heel. If you look at your heel, the skin will probably look distinctly red and sore.

Unfortunately, the wedding includes a dance and you are stuck for the whole evening with these very pretty, but now very painful, shoes. That night you finally get home and, with a great sigh of relief, are able to remove the offending objects. You now have a large blister on your heel. You have just experienced the various stages of inflammation. Had you taken off the shoes, at the first twinge of soreness, with just the slight redness of the skin where you had inflamed a patch of skin cells, then the skin would have quickly returned to normal. The redness, indicating an increased blood supply in response to the irritation, would have allowed the body to operate its repair mechanism. The longer it was inflamed, the longer it will take to return to normal.

Now let's look at the blister. The skin over the fluid of the blister is probably going white. The fluid has built up to protect the tissues underneath the skin. I am afraid you have killed the skin and it will eventually fall off. If, as probably happened, you wore the shoes too long, and the blister burst while you were dancing the night away, you may start to get some thickening of the tissues underneath. It may get so hard as to form a corn that you then have to shave off.

If you can keep in mind those three levels of inflammatory response, then that is all the pathology that you really need to understand the nature of lower back pain. Our bodies are pretty amazing concoctions. The more you understand them, the easier it is to make the right responses to help them.

---

### THE THREE STAGES OF INFLAMMATION

- A little inflammation, a simple reddening of the skin, it gets better of its own accord. The longer the reddening, then the longer the time to heal.
- The blister indicates a bigger response in order to protect the tissues underneath. There was so much pressure on the surface skin that it died. It will get better but new skin will have to form under the old, and the old will fall off.
- Burst the blister and continue with pressure, and the body will harden the skin to form a thick corn. You will probably need to shave off the hard skin.

Armed with this understanding of inflammation we can start to apply it to the pressure of a bulging disc onto a nerve. The disc is the shoe, and the nerve is the skin. The nerve gets slightly reddened and inflamed. There may be a bit of an ache around the backside and along the back of the thigh, with some pins and needles further down into the calf muscles and maybe even into the foot. The symptoms are probably worse standing and sitting as the weight-bearing is causing the flat tyre to constantly bulge and exert pressure on the nerve. You will probably notice that while you are on the move the symptoms are easier to control. Though it will depend on the size of the bulge, you'll find there is less permanent pressure on the nerve when you are moving around than when you are in the fixed position of sitting or standing. Movement also improves circulation and therefore helps reduce the build-up of swelling. Less swelling, less pressure. Conversely, standing and sitting cause the disc to bulge even more, resulting in more pressure, more inflammation and more pain.

## STRAIGHT TALKING ABOUT BED REST

Just as fashion trends seem to follow an invisible signal that suddenly invokes a collective response, so too has 'bed rest' as a treatment. Forty or fifty years ago the treatment of choice for any back pain, no matter its cause, was two weeks' bed rest. Today, it's generally active movement and no bed rest, the perceived wisdom being that the healing process is better served main- taining good movement and good muscle tone.

Muscle tone is really the natural tension in a muscle at rest. It is a sensation in a muscle of its alertness to perform. It should not be too hard and tense nor too soft and flabby. I have had the privilege of treating many Olympic athletes whose muscular structures are at a stage of honed perfection. There is a wonderful sense of impending action in them. They are ready to respond at the sound of the gun.

You can get a sense of this for yourself by first feeling your biceps muscle in the front of the forearm. Feel how soft it is but at the same time how it pushes against your pressure on it. Now, in a sitting position, reach behind and feel the muscles running parallel to each side of the lumbar spine, the erector spinae muscles. These are at the moment actively keeping you upright in your chair. Again this is all down to our old friend proprioception. The erector spinae muscles are balancing you in space. Nerves sensitive to your balance in space are actively, every millisecond, signalling to your brain. Your brain is responding with signals to your erector spinae to keep you upright. Hence, that sense of active awareness in the muscles. This is the sensation of resting muscle tone.

If you lie down too much, those muscles keeping you upright against gravity are not being stimulated and will very quickly lose that active awareness. This will make you more vulnerable to injury by not being ready to respond. So, certainly too much bed rest for the wrong condition will not help you to get better quickly. On the other hand, if you have a badly bulging disc, with pressure on a nerve, then a few days' bed rest to reduce the bulging pressure can bring magical relief. Just because the pendulum swing of fashion favours active exercise doesn't mean that bed rest was wrong. Just choose the right treatment for the right problem.

# 5 THE USER-FRIENDLY GUIDE TO UNDERSTANDING YOUR BACK

Back pain, or back problems, are really about two ends and a middle.

- *Lower back problems* are about coping with standing upright. They're about attempting to balance the performing seal on stilts while continually squashing our discs with the force of gravity.

- *Upper back problems* are about how we attempt to cope, or not, with the world around us. About the problems that arise from too many hours sitting at a desk, posturing to the PC, and about time spent in a car on motorways and in traffic jams. They're about sitting in a chair breast-feeding a baby at five o'clock in the morning.

- *The middle back* is different again. The middle is about posture.

If you're sitting in a chair at the moment it's a pretty good bet that you'll be sitting slumped with the middle of your back curved out, backside near the front of the chair and your shoulders rounded. Your back is like a 'C' curve, from the sacrum, right through your spine to where the base of your head meets your neck.

Now wriggle your backside as far back in the chair as you can. Notice how immediately you begin to be more upright. Next run a finger down the front of your chest bone – the sternum – to where it ends, about five inches above your navel. Next make your spine push forward towards that finger. You should be able to feel the end of your breastbone pushing against your finger.

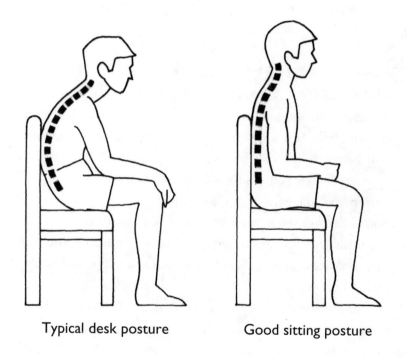

Typical desk posture          Good sitting posture

Did you notice at the same time how your whole chest lifted forward, and the shoulders came back and down – instead of being scrunched up towards your ears? Also, if you did it properly, you should have felt your neck straighten and a sense of lightness from your lower back to the base of your skull. That one action, changing the shape at the middle of your back, completely alters the posture in the neck and lower back, putting them into a neutral position.

Try to get a feel of your own body; most of our problems would be solved if we became more aware of our shells. For a moment, slump in the worst way, then do the exercise just described. Sense the difference and then try to use the latter position more when you're sitting. We could make the tasks of either end of the spine easier if we were to exercise just a little control over the middle.

## PASSIVE POSTURAL PROGRAMMING (PPP)

All day and every day you are passively programming your own personal biological computer (PBC). Passive Postural Programming, PPP for short, is loading your personal settings. It's memorising your habits so that your posture can be repeated and set with the necessary muscle patterns instilled in your hard drive.

That was fine when you wanted to learn to walk and instil in your hard drive the integrated circuits that now run 'walk mode'. Unfortunately you didn't want to imprint indelibly into your circuits that awful shape that you adopt for those hours hunched over the other computer!

If you don't want to become the victim of PPP you need have to take active steps to avoid it. You have to perform Active Postural Programming. You have to learn to click out of 'desk-sitting mode' and click on to 'upright mode'. It doesn't matter if you are just sitting back from your desk or about to stand up. There is one very simple input signal that you can give to your

PBC. In fact it is so simple that you will wonder why you have never done it before. But you must be consistent and do it every time you come away from 'desk sitting mode' for it to be effective. I can promise you profound change if you do. All you have to do, preferably standing up, is put your hands behind your back, interlock your fingers, and pull your shoulders back. Try to feel your shoulder blades meet at the back and your chest open out in front of you. You need only do it for five seconds. That's enough time to 'click off' one mode and engage another. It's as simple as that. The only difficult thing is to remember to do it.

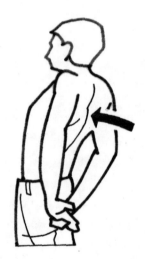

Shoulder blades meeting
behind the back

What most people do, that leads to a lifetime of postural pain, is to run 'desk mode' while they are standing upright. They stand up with the upper back still slumped over an invisible desk, merely curving in at the lower back and neck to assume some semblance of an upright posture.

We can normally run lots of programmes simultaneously on our screen but it seems that we can't run two postural programmes at the same time. This is why we must definitively click one off and deliberately engage another. Make a vow today to always take five seconds to click off one programme and engage another, for instance when standing up from sitting. The rewards are greater than the sum of the parts.

# 6 THE UPPER BACK

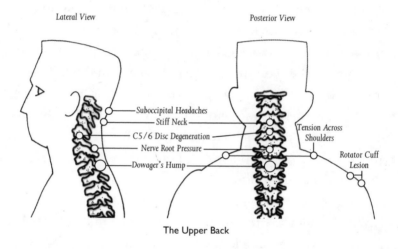

Lateral View          Posterior View

Suboccipital Headaches
Stiff Neck
C5/6 Disc Degeneration
Nerve Root Pressure
Dowager's Hump
Tension Across Shoulders
Rotator Cuff Lesion

The Upper Back

If standing up caused problems for a lower back, then the upper back, when we sit, is where the human animal really meets the world that we've created from our survival of the economically fittest. We have been standing, walking, running, in various stages of uprightness, for more years than we could name. It's only in the last few seconds, in evolutionary time, that we have sat down to truly become the victims of the environment we have created. If we haven't fully evolved to standing then we certainly haven't even begun to evolve to sitting. Hence the plethora of problems that this brings. Posture is always our confrontation with gravity. And sitting at a desk puts us in a special postural situation; I call it the desk-sitter's disease, the computer crouch or PC posture.

## DESK-SITTER'S DISEASE

Forty years in central London, attending the ills of the inhabitants of this city, have shown me just about all the variations possible for this condition. Because it's less dramatic than lower back pain, and necessitates less absenteeism from work, it's less statistically recorded. Even if you manage to avoid major incidents of lower back pain, you are unlikely to escape some of the symptoms of 'desk-sitter's disease', whether it's only aching across the shoulders from too long surfing the Internet or driving on the motorway. It attacks young and old, male and female without discrimination. In fact the young, more addicted to the computer, are the new sufferers from its bite, as they hunch for hours over their computer screens. So they begin, earlier than their parents, a lifetime's confrontation with this modern instrument of slow torture.

It's not just the unnatural position one adopts in front of the computer but more the inordinate amount of time spent there.

The computer, miracle though it undoubtedly is, is also something of a time waster. Some companies have started imposing a ban on the use of inter-departmental emails, because of their cost in time and money to production. Instead of staff sending emails to each other they are being encouraged to meet face to face or contact by telephone.

Though the reasons for this directive are a cost-saving exercise there will be hidden benefits as well. Any time away from 'computer crouch' is worthwhile. Getting up and talking to your colleagues, or telephoning them, at least gives space and time away from your PC posture. Time to straighten up, shrug the shoulders and reset your own musculo-skeletal PBC settings.

The accumulated moments, away from the desk and the

computer, will add up over the 50 years from school to retirement to a princely sum. If these moments can be used to shrug the shoulders; arch backwards with the spine; turn the neck from side to side and flex the chin forward to stretch the back of the neck, it will make a massive contribution to preventing the full ramifications of desk-sitter's disease.

Prevention is always better than cure, so let's look at what the presentations of desk-sitter's disease are and how best to deal with them. As the computer dominates all our lives I will use some computer language. Most of us are familiar with 'www' as the symbol for the world wide web; I am going to use it to introduce all of the problems relating to our musculo-skeletal systems. Though in this case 'www' will stand for:

- What is it?
- Why is it?
- What can you do about it?

## WWW. TENSION ACROSS THE SHOULDERS

### WHAT IS IT?

This is very simple. It's that sense of tightness across the shoulders that all of us have felt from time to time. It may be from studying for exams, driving the car on a motorway in pouring rain or more likely just sitting at the office desk. Whatever the cause, it still hurts the same.

## WHY IS IT?

The neck is like the jib of a crane, angled forward, with the head as the load. The muscles attached to the upper ribcage run alongside the neck to the base of the skull. They have to hold the head in a fixed position, which leads to severe tension on the attachments to the upper ribcage.

Remember, muscles that are contracting use energy in the form of glycogen obtained from the blood supply. One of the waste products of this process is lactic acid. Normally muscles work on an on/off basis, continually contracting and relaxing. As we've seen, they don't comfortably cope with being contracted for long periods of time.

Arteries, the tubes coming from the heart, have muscular walls so that they can constrict or dilate to pump blood into an area. Veins don't have muscular walls, so they can't pump. They rely either on gravity or on the repetitive action of muscular contraction and relaxation, for blood to be drained along them. Tense, contracted muscles squeeze the veins, which interrupts normal drainage. The result is that lactic acid doesn't get drained away but seeps into the substance of the muscles, where it excites nerve endings and causes pain.

When you run up – or in my case, walk up – a flight of stairs, and find the front of your thighs burning, that's lactic acid building up too quickly for your circulation to disperse it. The best thing is to wait, panting for a few moments, at the top of the stairs to allow time for your circulation to catch up and clear it.

Though similar, shoulder pain is usually not so acute but lasts longer as it's caused by the muscles not being used in an on/off manner. Muscle fibres gradually become hardened, and painful to touch, from the lactic acid deposited in them. Hence the very tender feeling if somebody squeezes you across the top of the shoulders, and the hard, ropy feel of the muscle tissue.

A similar problem is experienced after several hours driving a car at night, perhaps with the windscreen wipers barely clearing the heavy rain, the oncoming dazzling light on the wet glass, as you sit tensely focused on the road ahead, your shoulders and neck set in a fixed position. There must be few people reading this book that have not at some time felt its bite.

## WHAT CAN YOU DO ABOUT IT?

There is a very easy answer. Don't let it happen in the first place.

I am always trying to persuade my patients to do what I call a 'waiting for the kettle to boil exercise'. That means something you can do at any time of the day. It may be while waiting to decide the next word to write. It may be listening to someone talking to you on the telephone. It may be literally waiting for the kettle to boil. Whatever, whenever, just use those golden moments that are present every day for all of us.

There's one very simple 'waiting for the kettle to boil' exercise that you must adopt as a habit until it becomes imprinted in your hard drive.

### Keep shrugging your shoulders

This is one of the simplest but most effective things that we all need to do, but it's important to get it right. You can do it standing or sitting. All you do is shrug your shoulders up to your ears, while letting your arms hang loosely – never lift the arms up sideways just let them hang totally limp by your sides. What you are doing is simply pumping blood supply through the muscles;

the more often you do it the better. This simple, always available remedy is just about the best return for investment you can ever make.

The only trouble is, once the muscles have become too hard, it doesn't work and you may need some deep and rather painful massage to squeeze and stimulate blood supply along the now congested, hardened channels. The best thing is not to let it get to this stage. When you first start working in an office environment do the shoulder-shrugging exercise to prevent the problem developing. Have your screen so that you are forced to sit upright, and try not to hunch your shoulders. Don't forget when you stand up to put your hands behind the back, interlock the fingers, and pull the shoulder blades back to meet each other. You only have to do it for five seconds. Surely even you, with your impossibly busy schedule, can find five seconds! This one must become indelibly printed in your personal biological computer (PBC) so that it becomes second nature.

## WWW. SUB-OCCIPITAL HEADACHES AND TENSION

### WHAT IS IT?

The 'occiput' is the name of the bone at the base of the skull where the head fits on the top of the spine. There are complicated sets of muscles that are attached from the occiput to the top of the spine. They move the head on the spine and, more to the point, hold it still for hours on end. These muscles are one of the very common sources of tension and pain.

## WHY IS IT?

This is very similar to shoulder tension and for much the same reasons. Imagine you're driving in the rain at night staring at the oncoming headlights with your head in a fixed position. You all know what the back of your neck feels like in this situation, and that's from just a few hours. Multiply this by the hours at a desk spent looking at a screen and you can imagine why this area can become so painful. Again the pain is due to the build-up of lactic acid in the muscle tissue.

Sadly, it seems, we haven't yet developed a natural mechanism to cope with our modern environment. Our structures, and their function, lag behind the demands we put upon them, so we must instead rely on our own efforts for relief. Once more the evolution of our structure hasn't matched the evolution of our ideas.

## WHAT CAN YOU DO ABOUT IT?

There are several simple things you can do to prevent and relieve the symptoms.

- Again, to begin with, the only *sure* way is to avoid getting in this situation in the first place. Keep the head mobile and in a neutral position.
- The next simple measure, though not while driving, is from time to time to straighten up in your chair so that your neck is upright, and then let you head drop forward, with the chin trying to touch the chest. See how you move all the structures under the base of the skull. This simple move stretches the sub-occipital muscles and helps increase blood supply and pump the venous drainage. You can do this when you are

driving by letting your head gently drop forward. This allows the back of the neck to be stretched, permitting a little more blood to flow to the starved sub-occipital muscles.

■ Next try dropping your neck forward, as far as it will comfortably go, and now gently rotate the head from side to side, while the back of the neck is stretched out by the weight of the head hanging forward.

■ Now (not to be attempted when driving) stand up, put your hands behind your back and try to make your shoulder blades meet at the back. This will not only keep the circulation going but will help to stop PC posture from getting established. As you pull the shoulder blades back feel how your chest opens up. This expansion improves your heart's function and increases venous and lymphatic drainage.

■ Still standing, shrug the shoulders up and down a few times, and then let the neck drop fully forward, head hanging down, chin to throat, and again rotate the head a few times. This is a must when you have a chance to stand up at the petrol station – a perfect 'waiting for the kettle to boil' moment.

Have a go at all these moves and see how they work. They are very simple but very effective. Those few golden, between tasks, moments will reset your circulation and help the rest of the journey.


## WWW. C5, C6 DISC DEGENERATIVE CHANGES

### WHAT IS IT?

Quite simply it's the neck wearing out a bit. It may not hurt at all or it may give rise to bouts of acute pain and stiffness and, although at most times these will disappear of their own accord, they can be alarming. Knowing what's going on will help.

## WHY IS IT?

I'm now going to give you another powerful piece of user-friendly information. Earlier I asked you to focus on moving your head on the top of the spine; now I want you to feel how the neck moves. Put the flat of one hand behind your neck, as far down as you can, to roughly where the shoulders start to slope away from the spine, then gently bend the neck backwards and forwards. You should notice that nearly all the movement seems to happen at one place, that place is, counting from above down, at the level of the 5th and 6th neck bones, of the cervical vertebrae. The powerful muscles under the base of the skull and top of the neck effectively block that area from moving. Similarly the shoulders meeting across the base of the neck, and the tension across the top of them, limits free movement at this level.

In this situation the only place available for movement is at the base of the neck at the level of the C5 and C6 vertebrae. So it's no surprise that this is the bit of the neck that usually wears out first. It's like taking a piece of metal and instead of 'bowing' it you just bend it at one spot. You eventually get metal fatigue.

The neck is not metal but made of bone and disc, joined by ligaments and moved by muscles. The discs are the flexible parts and so it is they that, when overworked, fail first. Imagine the number of times, in the course of each day, that the disc at this C5/C6 bending point is operated. Remember that discs are like car tyres, blown up with fluid not air, and the outer casing, called the annulus, is the tyre wall. Picture the years of repeatedly bending, backwards and forwards and side to side and think of the gradual wear to this tyre wall. As it weakens, fluid inside the disc is gradually squeezed out through the overstretched and weakened outer wall, eventually leading to a flat tyre. Now a flat tyre is unstable and dangerous. Flat discs are just the same; they are unstable and dangerous.

## WHAT CAN YOU DO ABOUT IT?

I regret to say that wear and tear changes are pretty inevitable given our postural patterns. But what one can do is try to delay the onset and minimise the effects. As the buckling effect is due to the tension under the base of the skull and across the top of the shoulders, it's really about making sure that those areas are as relaxed as possible. The remedy is to be constantly aware of preventing the build-up tensions at those vulnerable areas, under the base of the skull and across the top of the shoulders.

- Never forget to 'click off' desk mode, and always remember to engage 'upright mode' on your PBC, when you stand up from the desk or chair (see page 56).
- Regularly shrug your shoulders up and down and then let them relax.
- Drop the chin to the front of the throat to stretch the head forward on the top of the neck.
- Take regular breaks.

These are very simple measures, and yet the rewards are enormous.

## WWW.STIFF NECK

### WHAT IS IT?

You have probably had an episode of it already. You may have woken up with a painful stiff neck, or, surprisingly it could be triggered by drying your neck with a towel. Whatever the cause, you are suddenly painfully restricted and have to turn your whole body to look behind you. The first time it happens it can be really alarming. Fortunately it will usually disappear in a few days.

### WHY IS IT?

Apart from in later years, when accumulated wear and tear leads to stiff joints in the neck, most episodes of stiff neck are due to muscle spasm or guarding (tightening up). We need to go back to the explanation earlier, of how the nerve endings, through the controlling muscles, balance you and carefully organise the movement of one vertebra on another.

One day, in an unguarded moment, as a result of towelling your neck or lying too long in one position, the ligaments joining one vertebra to the next are overstretched. The nerve endings fire up the signal to the brain, the signal is not recognised, and you register, 'You have performed an illegal operation and will be shut down.' Without further warning, muscles guard, go into spasm, and produce an acute stiff neck.

There are few of us human animals that will not experience this in our lifetime. If you're unlucky, once this instability is there, it may happen with annoying regularity. Perhaps the first thing to say, though, is that it will usually go of its own accord. The body has gone into a sudden state of chaos instead of order, but, fortunately, it has the propensity to return to normal. We possess the innate ability to, as it were, re-boot the system back to the factory settings.

## WHAT CAN YOU DO ABOUT IT?

- Take some painkillers and/or anti-inflammatories. Your doctor can prescribe those. These will help, in that limiting the pain reduces the body's automatic protective mechanism of muscle guarding. Anti-inflammatories, such as ibuprofen, will reduce the reactions of inflammation that the body sets up to protect you from what it perceives to be a potentially damaging moment.

- Wear a soft cervical collar. This is a great help. A cervical collar is muslin wrapped round a spongy material, with a Velcro fastening, that can be wrapped round the neck to support it. By supporting the neck you let the muscles relax, and convince your body's computer to restore order out of chaos.

- Do some shoulder shrugging. Also maintaining some gentle movement, in the relatively painless directions, will speed recovery. It might feel very painful at the time but it *is* temporary.

- An ice-pack is also worth trying, particularly in the very acute initial stages. Frozen peas from the deep-freeze will do fine. Wrap them in a thin towel or serviette (don't put directly on the skin as ice can 'burn'), and place on the painful area.

- Apply some heat. If the condition has been there for a few days you may find that warmth is more beneficial. Try an old towel soaked in hot water and then wrung out. Place it over the back of your neck and it will help increase the blood supply. In principle, ice is to reduce swelling in an acute condition and heat is to help improve blood supply in a more established problem.

## WWW.NERVE ROOT PRESSURE

### WHAT IS IT?

This can vary from a mild aching at the side of the neck radiating to one shoulder, to an almost unbearable neck pain and severe toothache-like pain into the arm and hand. The technical name for this is 'brachial neuritis'. Brachial means arm, and neuritis means nerve inflammation.

People who get pain radiating towards one shoulder and down into the hand usually have a history of recurrent episodes of stiff neck in the past. Typically they assumed that those episodes were normal. They weren't, those episodes were usually early warning signs of a future problem.

Though a disc may be pressing on a nerve in the neck, as it emerges from the spinal cord, the pain is generally felt in the arm and hand. It's the same as hitting your funny bone at the elbow; the tingling is felt along the course of the nerve to the relative fingers. So, where you feel the pain will depend on which disc level, and therefore which nerve, is affected.

The C5/6 disc will usually affect the thumb and index finger. The nerve, from this level, is called the radial nerve and, in the neck, is probably the most common one to be affected. You may get anything from complete numbness to a mild tingling. You will probably also get considerable pain in the upper back, on that side, and sometimes pain radiating to the whole of the arm.

Sadly bedtime will bring little relief. Your circulation slows down at night, so swelling builds up. If you have been lucky enough to get to sleep you may well be woken at about 4 a.m. with intense, unremitting pain. Our circadian rhythms – our time balance with the solar system – reach their lowest ebb at about four in the morning. Circulation, and with it our potential immune system response, is at its lowest. Our systems are unable to respond to problems. This is all likely to have been caused by a simple 'flat tyre'.

## WHAT CAN YOU DO ABOUT IT?

The body's self-repair mechanisms have been overwhelmed and are temporarily unable to cope with the situation. So don't panic too much; just try a bit of damage-limitation control.

- Painkillers, anti-inflammatories and a cervical collar will definitely help.
- Try some shoulder shrugging, bending the neck forward, and gentle rotation from side to side.
- Put one hand on top of your head. The curious thing, as many people have found, is that putting one hand on the top of your head, instead of hanging it down by your side, usually helps and can be a godsend in helping to get to sleep at night. By doing this, you are effectively shortening the nerve and therefore reducing the pull over the bulging disc. Conversely, dragging the arm down, while carrying a briefcase or hand-bag for example, usually increases the pain. If the four o'clock in the morning scene has hit don't try to stay in bed and fight it. However badly it may be hurting, and though you're

reluctant to leave the comfort of your warm bed, you're much more likely to relieve the symptoms if you get up and take a walk around, with your hand on the top of your head to reduce the 'drag' on the nerve root. You can also try shrugging the shoulders to kick-start your flagging circulation into action.

### X-rays and MRI scans

If the symptoms persist, and particularly if the thumb is numb, go and see your doctor. He or she may advise some MRI scans or x-rays. These are worthwhile as they may help to eliminate the rare occasions when there is some more serious underlying pathology. However, do remember, when the symptoms have gone, the scans or x-rays will probably look exactly the same. All that happened was that the chaos resolved; order was restored and the symptoms stopped.

The real problem, chaos, that is the direct cause of the symptoms, doesn't actually show on the pictures. Chaos is a dynamic state. X-rays and MRIs are like photographs. They are static pictures of a moving structure and cannot, therefore, depict an active process. They merely record a frozen moment in time.

I often explain this to patients, by pointing out that if we were to have five sets of scans from five patients, with varying degrees of symptoms, from agonisingly acute pain to symptom-free, then put the pictures on the screen and invite a consultant to match the patient to the pictures, it would only be chance that he could identify the patient by the picture. The worst symptoms, at the time, might have the best pictures with seemingly nothing to show. Conversely, the mildest symptoms can often present with the most horrific-looking pictures. It is what has happened to the dynamic equilibrium – that state that we are normally in all the time and take for granted – that determines symptoms and this cannot be shown on a static picture. It is really important to take that on board, as it is the key to understanding virtually all ills, particularly any involving the musculo-skeletal system.

## Prevention

Preventing the incident from happening again cannot be guaranteed, but it's definitely worth trying. Since the problem is the unstable (flat tyre) disc, what we need to do is to protect it from further instability. Posture is probably the most important factor in this.

It would be rare to find someone with a nerve root problem who did not have other factors present as well. If you have one area, the C5/C6 level of the vertebrae for example, that is over-mobile and therefore unstable, you will inevitably have some levels, above and below, that don't move enough.

The upper back and neck, in providing all the various ranges of movement available, is an integrated team effort. Ideally each vertebral unit, or wobble-board section, should have a full range of movement, and if each unit were to work normally then the problem wouldn't happen in the first place. So it's important to heed any warning signals. If you have already had neck problems, then the following tips can help reduce the likelihood of further incidents.

■ Try to sit more upright; shrug the shoulders up and down; then bend the head forward to stretch the base of the neck. What you're trying to do is get more units into normal action to spread the workload. In a desk-bound world there is hardly a person I have seen who does not have some blocking of movement in the vertebrae between the shoulder blades. Though this is a difficult area to get at, the rewards for encouraging more movement here are really worthwhile.

- Do the 'making the shoulder blades meet at the back; exercise. Make it a habit, when you get up from sitting at a desk, to always stand up and put your hands behind your back, as if trying to make the shoulder blades meet. As you do this, feel the chest opening up. It's not the 'forced action, shoulders back, chest out, army parade' command, but something much more subtle. All you need to do is reach behind your back, at roughly bra strap level – come on guys use your imagination – and push gently in so that the middle of your back straightens up. It's very simple, very gentle and extremely effective.

Stand up and try it now. Remember, it's not a strong muscular contraction; it's merely changing your centre of gravity. Think of someone pushing you in at that level; the rest changes automatically.

## WWW.DOWAGER'S HUMP

### WHAT IS IT?

This is the rather unattractive bump that some women develop in the spine across the top of the shoulders. It may be quite painless or it may feel sore and uncomfortable. The trouble is that it forces the area above it, in the lower part of the neck at the vulnerable C5/6 level, to curve in the opposite direction to compensate. The name derives, supposedly, from a slightly overweight dowager duchess who used to support the weight of her pearl necklace by hunching forward. That image may be a thing of the past, but the condition is very much one of the present.

## WHY IS IT?

You don't have to be a dowager duchess to suffer by sitting for hours at the computer. Like so many conditions, there can be many causes, but a large bust can be a real handicap – just ask any woman who has had to support one for years. Let's look at the applied mechanics.

### Big bust back

- Everything hangs from the spine.
- The spine is at the back; the bust is in the front.
- Just look at the side-on profile, and see how far the bust is in front of the spine.
- In a heavy woman it is probably a good ten inches or so from the spine.
- If each breast were just one kilogram (2.2lb) in weight, to stop the spine bending forward, there would have to be a constant counteracting force, pulling backwards, of 20 kilograms (at least 40lb).

### Other complications

So, day in, day out, your back will have a compression force, focused between the shoulder blades, resisting that forward weight. No wonder women suffer. As well as dowager's hump, this can result in neck tension, pain between the shoulder blades or sub-occipital headaches. The structures involved – upper back,

across the shoulders, lower neck and under the base of the skull –
become so entrenched and the muscles so irritable from the
constant abuse, that rightly the sufferer comes to dread another
day in front of a computer screen.

## WHAT CAN YOU DO ABOUT IT?

These are some practical things to do to help.

- Make sure you have a suitable supportive bra.
- Make sure the straps over the shoulder are broad as they are
  inclined to cause deep ridges in the tissues across the top of
  the shoulders. This can not only be painful but it can affect
  the nerves coming from the neck to the arm. This area is
  called the brachial plexus.
- Make sure also that there is a broad band at the back, as this
  can help ease some of the pain between the shoulder blades.
- Frequently do the 'making the shoulder blades meet behind
  the back' exercise.
- Keep shrugging the shoulders to keep the muscles exercised
  and maintain the blood supply to these overworked tissues.
- Try exercising with one of those large Swiss balls pushing
  against your middle and upper back, so that you can arch
  backwards over the ball. That can really help ease the pain at
  the end of the day.
- A heat pad over the upper back can help the circulation.
- You can also get help from acupuncture, physiotherapy,
  cranio-sacral therapy, chiropractic, osteopathy and massage.

Above all, don't let it build up; nip it in the bud early on.

## WWW.MOUSE USER'S MALADY (MUM)

### WHAT IS IT?

This is a relatively new condition as the computer mouse has been with us for only a few years, but its impact on our lives is enormous. It is probably already the single biggest cause of repetitive strain injury (RSI) from pain in the forearm, tendonitis at the wrist, rotator cuff syndrome to chronic pain in the side of the neck. It is also the single biggest contributor to the problems of the upper back.

### WHY IS IT?

The trouble is it's virtually impossible to control the mouse without:

- Getting tense in the back of the forearm.
- Raising the shoulder to the side of the neck.
- Making the shoulder blades migrate laterally.

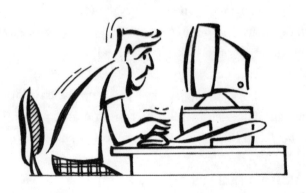

MUM and repetitive strain injury

A few years ago you couldn't pick up a magazine without reading an article about RSI. Some people vehemently claimed it didn't exist, while others sought damages from their employers for contracting it. I certainly think it exists; but it's an old problem with a new name. Let me give you a working idea of what happens.

It relates to the muscles needing to be used on an on/off basis rather than constantly contracted. In our earlier years of evolution we were a much more active animal. Like any other creature on the planet, our musculo-skeletal structures were always on the move. The tasks we undertook meant frequent movement and the constant contraction and relaxation of muscles.

Our intellect, however, has far outpaced our purely animal side. The animal side cannot cope with the demands put upon it, given our existing physical and functional settings. We can't simply access the 'settings' or 'active desk top' menu on our body's computer to instantly change our operating procedures. Any changes in our basic response mechanisms have to come about through evolutionary change.

We need to evolve structurally to cope with this world that our intellect has created. The problem is that, intellectually, we are moving the goalposts too fast for the necessary structural changes of evolution to catch up. The symptoms that we suffer from are merely the inability of our bodies to cope with the unrealistic demands that we are putting on them.

## WHAT HAPPENS WHEN YOU USE A MOUSE

We trouched on this briefly in the opening chapter but, as it is so fundamental to our everyday existence, let's take another look.

When you look at the computer screen, and you are holding the mouse, you then decide to click to activate the cursor on some part of the screen. Almost at the speed of light, a chemical reaction zaps along the nerve – like igniting a dynamite fuse. *A nerve is like the fuse where flame zaps along at an incredible pace.*

Between the thought starting in the brain the nerve impulse has to 'relay' at several junction boxes, called synapses, before finally a tiny electrical impulse stimulates the muscle fibre to contract.

The stronger the impuse, the more fibres are stimulated and the stronger the contraction. Relay is the apt word, for, at each junction box (synapse), a special chemical called a neurotransmitter, is the 'baton' that bridges the gap and thus transmits the signal on its path to the muscle fibre. For a millisecond after that reaction, the chemical has to re-form to be ready to pass on another impulse. Now if you keep firing continuously, instead of some of the microscopic muscle fibres relaxing while they wait for their next ignition, they are constantly firing without a chance to recover.

Meanwhile the synapse burns in a permanent 'ignition' state so that you can no longer voluntarily command the muscle to relax. It's rather like having a screen saver to stop permanently etching an image on to the computer screen. You create a permanent pathway, along the nerve, from the brain to the brawn.

The result is the muscles along the back of the forearm are on continuous contraction, just like the muscles in the upper back and neck with the 'big bust back.' Lactic acid builds up in the muscle fibres and they become hard and tender.

Our machinery is made of masses of circuits that we control consciously, and subconsciously, via the brain, our central computer. Most of the time we are unaware of these circuits, for example our postural habit patterns. If we spend too long bending over the computer desk, so that we develop a bend forward at the middle of our thoracic spine, the area gradually becomes rigid as a permanent circuit is created. We then lose the ability to override the now fixed circuit, as we can no longer 'command' messages to that area.

Brilliant though the machine is, if we abuse it too much bits of it will break down and need repair. Thankfully, it is self-repairing. We cut ourselves and the skin heals, and normally within ten days you can barely see the repair. We fracture a bone, and over a few weeks, we create new bone to repair the fracture. Miraculous though this machine of ours is, having a knowledge of how it works, what goes wrong, how the body repairs it and what we can do to help, in both prevention and care, will enable us to suffer fewer problems.

## WHAT CAN YOU DO ABOUT IT?

The essential thing is to keep moving. If our environment dictates us to behave in a functionally harmful way it is up to us to be aware of the situation and take the responsibility for evasive action. But act we must if we are to avoid becoming a victim.

- As frequently as every five minutes, take your hand off the mouse and let your elbow rest on the desk. Now rotate your forearm a few times so that you get the benefit of both gravity drainage and muscular activity to break the build-up of an imprinted neuro-muscular circuit. Ten seconds is all that is needed, as long as it is done regularly.

■ Gently massage the forearm musculature to help the drainage mechanism.

■ Shrug the shoulders up and down a few times.

■ Consider using one of those wrist supports that allows you to support the wrist with less strain and contraction of the muscles of the forearm.

■ Always remember that it is better to prevent the build-up than to try to remedy the problem once it arises.

## WWW.TENNIS ELBOW

### WHAT IS IT?

It's a painful spot at the back of the elbow and sometimes radiating along the back of the forearm. You feel it when you grip with the hand, as in shaking hands, or even something as mundane as lifting a tea cup. It can be so painful that you drop the object in your hand. At its worst you may avoid shaking hands at all costs.

It is sometimes described as a strain of the common extensor tendon origin. That is the tendon that attaches all of the muscles along the back of the forearm to a small spot on the outside of the upper arm at the elbow.

### WHY IS IT?

Make a fist with your right hand while you feel with your fingers over the back of your forearm. Then clench and relax your fist a few times and feel the muscles contract and relax under your fingers. You are feeling the extensor muscles that bend, or extend, your hand backwards at the wrist. They are all attached to a small point on the back of the elbow the common extensor tendon origin.

When you play a backhand shot at tennis, or have your forearm extensor muscles continually contracted from controlling a mouse, you pull on the muscles where they are attached to the bone. Imagine the forces involved when you grip the racket and then hit and control a ball that now, with the length of the racket, is about a metre away from the point of attachment.

Bone is enveloped by a skin, called periosteum. The common extensor tendon attachment is on this periosteum, and a too-sharp pull, or a very prolonged one, can 'lift' the skin off the bone. This is extremely painful! It causes inflammation – the body's response to injury. It's like an open cut, deep inside. Every time you operate those muscles, the tendon attaching the muscle to this now loosened periosteum lifts it away from the bone. Each time you contract those muscles by playing a backhand tennis shot, shaking hands or even lifting a tea cup, you pull open the wound and prevent it from healing.

The body is a self-healing unit, but if you keep repeating the same injury eventually the healing mechanism stops trying. This is called a chronic problem; where the body has effectively stopped healing itself.

## WHAT CAN YOU DO ABOUT IT?

Of course the best thing to do is avoid getting it in the first place, but sudden injuries, like a bad backhand shot at tennis or a sudden strain when doing a spot of DIY, are impossible to guard against. Just be aware and take care. Slower injuries are potentially easier to deal with, though they have a habit of creeping up and becoming a problem before you realise it.

■ Don't stay too long holding the mouse. Every five minutes or so let go and just move your arm.

■ Try to relax your arm. Though this sounds easy in reality it's remarkably difficult to do. The best way is to keep making deliberate active movements involving the forearm.

■ Make a fist and then relax and repeat a few times.

■ Rest your elbow on the desk and rotate the forearm several times.

■ Use one of the forearm supports now available to rest on while you work.

■ Wear a tennis elbow support, the type that just grips the forearm below the elbow. This helps to stop the muscles pulling away from the bone.

■ Take frequent breaks.

## Homecare

You need to stimulate and encourage the body to heal itself.

■ Apply rubbing-in compounds. I particularly like Tiger Balm, available in most chemists, as it seems to create local heat and encourage blood supply.

■ Try an anti-inflammatory in gel form. Use this in the morning and before you go to bed at night. Just rub it in for about a minute.

■ A magnetic strip over the point of attachment of the tendon can also be very effective.

■ Hot and cold compresses also work well. Get a bowl of hot water and a bowl of cold and two flannels or old pieces of towel. Place the hot towel on the painful area for about 20 seconds, followed by the cold towel for 20 seconds. Alternate between hot and cold for fifteen minutes. This will help stimulate the circulation, improve blood supply and increase drainage, so it is worth doing.

### Further help

If you find that none of these measures seems to be helping it may be worth asking your GP to refer you to an orthopaedic specialist or rheumatologist. He or she will most likely give you a steroid injection. This can be very effective but, if you haven't dealt with the cause – the forearm muscle tightness – the problem may come back very quickly.

Sometimes a full plaster cast is necessary, worn for about a month, to fully immobilise the elbow and forearm to allow time for the periosteal damage to heal.

Surgery may also be necessary. The very severe, chronic problem occasionally requires that the tendon attached to the bone be attached to a new undamaged site. Big problems unfortunately sometimes need drastic solutions.

## WWW.TENDONITIS AT THE WRIST

### WHAT IS IT?

This is an acute pain felt on the front or back of the wrist due to an inflammation of the tendon and its sheath in the front or back of the wrist. It's useful to remember that any word ending in with 'itis' denotes inflammation. This 'itis' is a form of RSI. The pain and discomfort in operating the wrist may be so severe as to totally incapacitate. Any movement involving these tendons, or even holding the wrist in a fixed position, can be extremely painful. It is one of the worst presentations of repetitive strain injury and one of the most difficult ones to manage.

## WHY IS IT?

Tendons, especially over areas where there is a lot of movement, such as the wrist, run inside a sheath or tunnel. The outside of the tendon and the inside of the tunnel are bathed in body oil – synovial fluid – so that normally the movement is virtually frictionless.

Using a mouse, and repeating the movements, with tense muscles, time and time again, leads to an irritation of the lining of the sheath and tendon. This is called tendonitis. (It's like the blister on the heel from a new pair of shoes that are too tight, where the skin gets red and raw from being repeatedly used for the same movement in the tense situation.) It can be extremely painful, often described as broken glass on an open wound, and extremely difficult to cure.

## WHAT CAN YOU DO ABOUT IT?

As ever, take all possible precautions to avoid getting it in the first place.

■   Try using one of those cushioned supports for the forearm. If the forearm is not supported properly, then it's the muscles that have to hold it still while operating the fingers to control the mouse. Used properly, it will relax the forearm musculature and lessen the effect on the tendons of the repeated clicking movement with the index finger.

- Check out the latest gizmos. There are now a variety of devices, such as wireless mouses, and free-moving gadgets, to point at the screen, rather than the conventional fixed mouse.
- Do 'waiting for the kettle to boil' exercises. Don't get caught in one position for too long, keep mobile and keep taking breaks. Take your hand off the mouse, or away from the keyboard, and make a full range of movement with the wrist and elbow. Gently massage the muscles in the forearm to help limit the build-up of harmful lactic acid in the muscle tissues.

## Home care

- Hot and cold compresses – simple but effective.
- Anti-inflammatory gel. You can rub in at night and in the morning. You can use it during the day as well.
- Splint. Supporting the wrist at night with a suitable splint can be worthwhile.
- Voice-activated word processing. There are now some really good voice-activated software programmes that work at a level of worthwhile efficiency. I have several patients, who, in desperation, have resorted to them and now would not dream of going back to a manual keyboard and mouse. Try experimenting with one, before the condition develops. I did when typing most of this book.

Further help

Treatment to the forearm with gentle massage may help the circulation. Osteopaths or chiropractors will provide some treatment directly to the affected area, and also to the spine to affect blood supply. Acupuncture can also be effective.

In most cases that require professional treatment it is essential to have complete rest from what seems to have caused the problem. I regret to say that many of the cases I have seen never seem to recover. That's why, armed with some understanding of the problem, it is so important that you take responsibility for your own wellbeing.

There is a fuller explanation about osteopathy and chiropractic later in the book but a brief description now may be useful in these sections on problems and treatment. Osteopathy and chiropractic are very similar in many ways yet at their extremes there are marked differences. In both professions manipulation is the key element of the treatment, though it is a process that has many variations. In most instances, and certainly in the public's perception, manipulation means a forceful movement usually resulting in an audible click; in osteopathy what is called a high-velocity thrust. As a generalisation chiropractors tend to give shorter treatments, more frequently and with often just some high-velocity thrust adjustments. Osteopaths tend to have a longer treatment session, using more repetitive movements to a joint, and accompanied by varying massage techniques, as well as perhaps a high-velocity thrust manipulation.

I think it is fair to say that, particularly with the use of cranial osteopathic methods, osteopathy has a gentler and more widespread approach. Though in the treatment of musculo-skeletal conditions they will both treat the same problems but often appear to use quite different approaches.

It would be unwise of me to suggest a preference between the two professions, as it will often come down to the skills and ability of individuals as to who may offer the best service. Take advice from your own doctor, or from a friend who has had a good experience with a particular individual practitioner, and see for yourself.

There is one word of advice that I would offer and that is beware of any one who wants you to sign up, and pay in advance with discounts, for 36 or so treatments. I am always suspicious that this approach has more leaning to commercialism than professionalism!

## WWW.ROTATOR CUFF LESION

### WHAT IS IT?

This is frequently, and usually mistakenly, called frozen shoulder. The symptoms are pain and stiffness of the shoulder that prevents a full range of movement, usually in one particular direction. This is due to a tendonitis, an inflammation of one of the four tendons that control the movement of the arm at the shoulder joint. Together, and individually, they elevate and rotate the humerus – upper arm bone – in its socket on the shoulder blade (scapula). This can make trying to put an arm in the sleeve of a jacket, or reaching sideways for something very painful. When reaching across to the passenger side of the car, or to a bedside table, the pain can be so sharp as to make you cry out involuntarily. It is usually painful to lie on that side at night.

WHY IS IT?

The best way to explain the cause is to demonstrate how the shoulder works normally, and how it can't work normally if it operates from the wrong starting position. You can do this exercise sitting down but it's easier if you stand up.

- Stand as upright as possible so that your shoulder blades are behind you, rather than rounded and facing forward.
- Now, starting with the palm of your hand by your side, lift your right arm out sideways. Continue to lift the arm, making a long arc until your arm is fully vertical, almost with the upper arm against the side of your face. Assuming your shoulder is quite normal this should have been an easy pain-free movement.
- Now let yourself be round-shouldered, so that you can feel your shoulder joints pointing more to the front – the sort of position you are in when you are sitting bent over your computer.
- Raise the arm again and continue as before. You should find it more difficult, and probably more painful, to go through the movement and impossible to lift to the same height as before. That's the sort of round-shouldered posture that sitting at a desk for long periods of time produces.
- Now put yourself in the typical posture that arises when you start to operate a mouse. The mere process of looking at the screen, and reaching forward to hold the mouse, tends to produce a degree of round-shouldered posture. Unfortunately, the moment you take hold of the mouse and begin to use it, it is virtually impossible not to, at the same time, raise the upper ribs – the area between the side of your neck and the shoulder. Just try it.

- Next, keeping your shoulders rounded and the same elevation of the upper ribs, try again to lift the arm sideways. It's now even more difficult.
- In the same round-shoudered position, try lifting your arm up in front, following the direction that your shoulder faces. You will find you can do this easily.

These exercises demonstrate how we compromise the function of the shoulder through extended periods at our desks and computers. It's like having the front wheels of a car towed at the wrong angle – you would start wearing the tyres out. The same happens with the shoulder. By constantly trying to elevate the shoulder in this state, gradually – or sometimes sharply – the tendons, which are no longer running a straight line in their grooves, become inflamed and restrict the range of movement. As you lift the head of the arm bone (humerus), it has to pass under the arch of bone formed by your collarbone and part of the shoulder blade, with the tendons lying between them. If the tendon, in tendonitis, is swollen it becomes too thick to pass under the arch if you lift the arm to the side.

Lifting the arm straight up in front of you is usually OK, as it doesn't trap the tendon.

When you lie on that side at night you are lying on the inflamed tendon and that is why it's painful. When it's really acute, even lying on the good side causes the bad one to hang in a position that becomes painful as well. Unsurprisingly, it can be very sleep disturbing.

## WHAT CAN YOU DO ABOUT IT?

Taking steps to improve your sitting posture can help prevent future problems. Be very aware, when you're using the mouse, to avoid the round-shouldered sitting posture and the elevation of the upper ribs that lie between the side of the neck and the shoulder.

### 'Waiting for the kettle to boil' exercises

- Frequently get up from sitting. Stand up and, with your hands held behind your back, try to make the shoulder blades meet at the back.
- With the arms hanging loosely by your sides, shrug your shoulders up and down. You can shrug them straight up and down or roll them backwards and forwards – or both. Try to avoid pinching the tendon. Each time it hurts you are increasing the swelling on the tendon, and certainly don't try and force it into the painful range.
- Let the head of the humerus hang in its socket by deliberately focusing on relaxing the upper arm and allowing the weight of the arm to hang loosely. If your should is very sore at night and keeping you awake, then get up and do the following little exercise. You can also do it during the day.

---

### INSTANT RELIEF FOR A PAINFUL SHOULDER

Find a fairly heavy object. The perfect thing is an old-fashioned flat iron (those heavy irons that our grandmothers used before the electric ones of today), that are now some-times used as a doorstop. But any heavy object that you could hold comfortably in the hand will do. Standing, hold the object on your bad side, lean over to that side and, letting the weight drag your arm down, gently swing the arm backwards and forwards. The idea is to 'let go' at the shoulder joint so that the weight of the arm, and whatever you are holding, gives some traction through to the head of the armbone. The suction effect of this action helps to increase the circulation and relieve the pressure within the shoulder joint itself.

### Homecare

- Raid the bathroom cabinet for some anti-inflammatory gel. Rubbing it over the tendon can help reduce the pain. It is best to use it before going to bed so that the effects last through the night, and again first thing in the morning to help through the day.
- Hot and cold compresses (see pages 84–5) can also be good if you make time in the evening.

### Further help

Physiotherapy, osteopathy, chiropractic, and acupuncture can all offer relief. Often working on the spine and upper ribcage rather than on the affected shoulder can have a dramatic effect.

Some years ago I was teaching a group of physiotherapists in Vienna. I was talking about shoulder problems and particularly the rotator cuff lesion. We finished the discussion, and I said that after the lunch break I would demonstrate a particular technique to correct elevation of the first and second ribs, since this was critical to the correct function of the rotatator cuff mechanism.

We were walking out to the dining hall when one of my

students, a 36-year-old physiotherapist, asked if I could help her with a problem. After a skiing accident when she was 18, she had not been able, despite numerous treatments, to elevate her left arm above the horizontal. I was suitably reticent about such a long-term problem but agreed to use her as my model when demonstrating the technique later that afternoon.

When we were all in the classroom after lunch, I asked her to sit on the treatment table facing the class, with me behind her. I then made her demonstrate the range of movement, as described in the arm elevation exercise, and told the class her history.

On the right, she elevated perfectly, but on the left, as she had said, her arm would not rise beyond the horizontal. I told her she certainly did have elevation of the ribs on the left, but I had no idea, after this length of time, how it would respond to treatment.

After a few minutes gently playing with the musculature, I got her to lie on her tummy and performed a corrective manipulation to the first and second ribs. They moved – slightly to my surprise – with a loud crack, and very cleanly.

Not knowing what would happen, I got her to sit up and asked her to try again to elevate the left arm. She briefly, through habit, hesitated at the horizontal level but then continued the movement straight up until the arm was completely vertical, in line with the normal side.

The audience gasped, she cried in complete delight and disbelief, and I had a very attentive class for the rest of the afternoon.

So the moral of the story is if you have a bad shoulder and none of the suggested exercises helps, try a good osteopath. There are many cases that undergo unnecessary surgery that could be helped by sensible complementary medicine.

## WWW.WHIPLASH

Though this is not really in the same category as the other 'desk-sitter's disease' conditions, it is nevertheless a common problem of our everyday lives and certainly a condition of confrontation with the environment, the environment in this case being our crowded and dangerous roads.

### WHAT IS IT?

It is the serious – or potentially serious – damage caused to the neck when a car accident leads to a very stiff neck. It is frequently accompanied by a severe headache. There may often also be a sense of disorientation.

### WHY IS IT?

Many people are familiar with the scenario of how, perhaps being hit from behind when your own car is stationary, the sudden impact causes the body to move forward and the neck, relative to the rest of the body, to be thrown into violent extension. Since the head is relatively heavier than the neck, this leads to varying degrees of damage, depending on the force involved, to the ligaments and joints of the cervical spine. It can also happen in a head-on crash, when the head is initially flung forward and then jerks violently backwards.

There are many minor variations, depending on the angle at which the collision occurs, but the basic mechanism remains the same, with damage to the joint structures in the neck. The reason for its seriousness is the potential to damage the delicate joints at the base of the skull and, in the most severe cases, to actually sever the spinal cord with the resultant quadriplegia – a paralysis of all four limbs.

The headache can often be extremely painful as sometimes there is a stretch of the meninges – the outer covering of the spinal cord running up in the neck and into the cranium. The pain can be of the same degree as with meningitis, but the irritation is a mechanical one, rather than one induced by a viral or bacterial infection as in meningitis.

The disorientation comes from the sudden uncontrolled movement of the body. A colleague of mine once rather graphically described it by imagining what would happen to a bucket of water sitting on the passenger seat, in the same situation. The water would go everywhere. We are made of some 90 per cent per cent water, and our water and cells get thrown all over the place as well. In one sudden moment, our long-established spatial awareness is thrown into chaos, and we experience this disorientation.

## WHAT CAN YOU DO ABOUT IT?

- If you are in a car accident, and it has been a severe crash, you will need to go to hospital for a check-up and possibly an x-ray. It's best to err on the side of safety rather than being too cavalier about the whole thing.
- An ice-pack on the back of the neck is a very good initial treatment.
- Take some homeopathic arnica. This suggestion will be frowned upon in some circles, but I know of nothing better to deal with shock to the system that is caused by whiplash. Any good chemist will stock arnica, and many can suggest

the best strength to take. I recommend Arnica 30 pills. Take a couple, sucking them under the tongue until they dissolve. Initially I suggest you take them that same day, every couple of hours. The next two or three days you can take them just three times per day, remembering always to try to take them some time before or after eating or drinking. They have always worked very well for me, and for my patients, too.

- Wearing a soft cervical collar for a few days may help by supporting the bruised and irritable neck structures.

- Make sure you try to get a good night's rest. Try pinching your pillow into a butterfly shape so that it can offer good support for your neck.

- If the pain is severe, then taking some ibuprofen for a few days will be a great help.

- Try letting your head hang forward so that the neck is 'opened' at the back. This helps to separate the facet joints at the back of the neck that may have been bruised at the initial hyperextension movement, when they can impact on each other rather like buffers on a train, when it stops suddenly.

- Similarly, gently bending the neck from side to side may help to mobilise and 'oil' the facet joints.

- Though the neck is the most vulnerable structure in this problem, effects can be felt in the upper back, between the shoulder blades, and even down into the lumbar spine. For some people the condition will swiftly resolve itself; for others symptoms can persist for many months, even years. Physiotherapy, osteopathy and chiropractic can all treat these problems and usually speed up the process of repair.

# 7 THE LOWER BACK

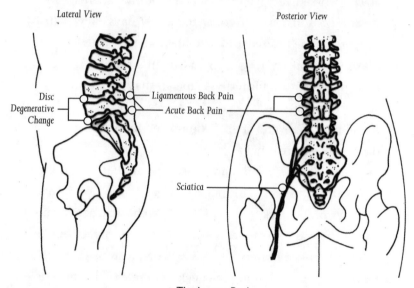

Lateral View                    Posterior View

Disc Degenerative Change — 
Ligamentous Back Pain — 
Acute Back Pain — 
Sciatica — 

**The Lower Back**

If problems in the upper back are predominantly the result of sitting, then it's the lower back that bears the brunt from standing upright. Animals, on all fours, carry the base of the spine, the sacrum, horizontally. In this horizontal position, the spine, with its sequential segments of vertebra-disc-vertebra, is wonderfully free and mobile. A vertical position, however, places a heavy toll on the function of the lower back.

It's really the discs, 'our car tyres', that have suffered from our upright evolution. The wear and tear changes to our discs are the underlying cause of virtually all lower back problems, as they don't yet seem to have evolved to cope with the demands we put on them.

## WWW.SIMPLE BACK PAIN

Simple, or ligamentous, back pain is the most common problem of the lot. It has become so common that we take it for granted, and have come to almost expect back pain as part of everyday life.

### WHAT IS IT?

Quite simply, it is a pain or ache in the back. It is usually worse in static positions such as standing, sitting or lying, and is generally relieved by walking and any active movements.

### WHY IS IT?

Since back pain generally improves when we are active and in muscular control, and worse when we are stationary and merely depending on our ligaments for support, this suggests the ligaments are the cause of the symptoms.

To give an example of ligamentous pain, try, while you are sitting, to rest your foot on a stool, so that the back of your knee is unsupported, allowing the ligaments at the back of the knee to be stretched. Within a few minutes, the back of the knee will start to ache, as the ligaments are put on unnatural stretch. That's ligamentous pain. That's the pain that the ligaments supporting the vertebrae give when you are standing still at a drinks party or in a supermarket queue. You keep fidgeting from one leg to

another in an effort to alleviate the strain on the relevant ligaments, which, without muscular control, are painfully attempting to support your whole body weight against gravity.

Think back to that image of the performing seal on stilts. We
have to balance on our two legs, with the spine, and the whole of
the upper body, supported by the sacrum between the two sides
of the pelvis at the sacroiliac joints. It's no wonder that the spine
rising vertically from the sacrum, through the bones and discs,
suffers from degenerative changes.

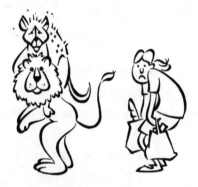

One of the imagines I use when teaching, to understand the
stress that's involved, is the Lion and the Hyena story. It
illustrates the problems of standing vertically and carrying
things. If I ask a group of students, 'How many times have you
seen a lion capture a hyena, kill it, stand up on its back legs, carry
the hyena across it shoulders and walk off into the jungle?' They
inevitably reply, 'Never.' But that is exactly what we do.

Of course the image of the lion with the hyena over its
shoulders is ridiculous, yet that's what we do virtually every day
of our lives. We get, metaphorically, cans of hyena from the
supermarket and walk back to our lair, laden down each side with
them. The spine, through the discs, is being daily compressed by

these loads. It's just as ridiculous for us to do it as it is for the lion. The lion hauls its prey along the ground; it wouldn't last long using our method of carrying.

If we weren't 'designed' to be upright, we certainly are not well adapted to standing and sitting, but at least we cope better on the move. Balancing upright requires a well-integrated feedback loop.

Let me explain. Feedback loops, as discussed in chapter 4, are at the heart of how we control our bodies and are one of the major reasons for dysfunction and pain. The loop is ligament→stretch receptor→nerve impulse→brain→nerve impulse→muscle. This loop is wonderful when we are on the move but not so hot when we are static. Ligaments, if you remember, have two functions. They are the leather retaining straps on a 'Mini' front door but with stretch receptors thrown in. One function is to stop you moving too far, the other is to provide proprioceptive signals to the brain to organise the muscles that control you.

Imagine that those leather retaining straps had stretch receptors that emitted a high-pitched whine the more you stretched them. If you were forcing open the door of the Mini, the more you pushed, the louder the whine would be. Well, that's what ligaments are and do. They emit a high-pitched whine in your brain, called pain, the more they are stretched.

When we stand or sit, we tend to slump without muscular support, making the ligaments responsible for all the weight-bearing. Ligaments are not designed to act in this way, and let you know by signalling pain. If you're standing, you start fidgeting from side to side, first leaning on one leg then the other desperately trying to take the load off the ligaments and stop the pain. The ligaments are not designed to be permanently stretched but merely, through their feedback function, to aid in organising muscle control.

## WHAT CAN YOU DO ABOUT IT?

There are many steps you can take to help prevent ligamentous back pain.

- Don't get into bad postural positions, such as lying on your tummy propped on your elbows reading a book, that will allow the ligaments to be stretched
- Try to avoid standing too long in one position – keep moving around.
- If you're sitting, put a cushion in the small of your back so that you are supported and balanced. This takes the strain off the ligaments.
- Posture is very important. When standing, try to balance in a neutral position, so that your weight is distributed on both legs, rather than on just one leg.
- Don't lift and carry more than you can help.

This last point is vitally important. We are all inclined, especially when we are young, to lift far too heavy weights. That single moment, whether it be lifting a heavy suitcase from a carousel or shifting a bulky piece of furniture, which leads to a ruptured disc, can be a disaster for the rest of your life. Today's problems are couched in yesterday's lifting.

### 'Waiting for the kettle to boil' exercises

By far the best is the 'two orifices' exercise. This exercise, more commonly known as the pelvic floor contraction, is the best return for investment that I know!

- Stand comfortably balanced on both legs. Now imagine you are desperately holding your bladder as hard as you can – there is a queue for the loo and if you're not careful it could be very embarrassing! At the same time, squeeze the cheeks of your backside together to try to avert a disaster!
- Hold this extreme contraction for about five seconds then let go of the tension by a half. Don't let go completely.
- You should now be standing with a nice sense of supporting your whole pelvic floor. More importantly, instead of your upper body being slumped into your spinal and pelvic ligaments, you are held by muscular control. There's an added bonus, too, it gives you a flatter tummy.

You can do this exercise standing, sitting, lying down or even on the move. The beauty of it is that nobody will even know what you are doing. It's a lifesaver. If you keep doing it you will gradually make it become your resting state position. By practising this simple technique regularly, and establishing it in your system, I guarantee that you will be able to prevent all your ligamentous lower back pain. It is that simple. All you have to do is keep remembering to do it!

## Homecare

You need to do everything possible to improve your feedback loop. You can't actively do anything to your ligaments as they are inert, but you can improve the response of the muscles to their signals. Ballet dancers who frequently sprain their ankles and need to get them back to perfect order for balancing, do the wobble-board exercise. Remember, that's standing on one leg on a breadboard over a tennis ball. As there are usually several dancers in a ballet class with the same problem, then they can do the balancing act and throw a tennis ball to each other at the same time. I don't recommend you do the same, but try the following:

- Stand balancing on one leg while you're at the washbasin, mirror, working in the kitchen – any place you can think of. Just get into the habit of balancing.
- Walk, walk, and walk. Walking is the single best everyday exercise that will help your back. It's easy, it's available, and it saves money! I don't care how you do it; walk to work, walk home, walk to the shops, walk the dog, walk up the stairs, even sleepwalk if you like. Just find every excuse to use this machine of yours in walk mode. What it does is integrate the whole of the performing seal on stilts and keep it at optimum working level.

## Further help

Ligamentous back pain is so common that I am afraid your doctor really is not going to be either sympathetic or particularly interested. There's nothing he or she can offer other than giving you analgesics, anti-inflammatories and suggesting exercise.

- Complementary medicine.

I would certainly look at Pilates or any good gym programme to help build up muscle tone. If yoga is your passion, be careful not to do too much hyperextension – that's bending backwards – it may stretch your ligaments even more, when it's muscle control that you need.

- Find a good osteopath or chiropractor. A common problem is having one leg that is longer than the other. This is usually caused by the sacrum becoming blocked asymmetrically between the two sides of the pelvis. This can be corrected by manipulating the sacrum between the ilia, and restoring normal leg length. This takes out the lateral instability and often enables the patient to balance better, which reduces ligamentous strain.

## WWW.LIGAMENTOUS BACK PAIN WITH DISC DEGENERATIVE CHANGE

### WHAT IS IT?

This is a little further down the line of wear and tear changes. Here, disc compression adds to the problem of an unnatural stretch of the ligaments. The symptoms are very much the same as ordinary ligamentous back pain but now you may notice more difficulty getting out of bed in the morning, and getting up from sitting down.

### WHY IS IT?

Again, the discs degenerating are the cause of the problem. Remember the idea of discs being like a car's tyres. A flat tyre is unstable; it can allow shear, as well as permitting the established controlled movements of flexion, extension, side-bending and rotation that we use to control our everyday movements.

As discs degenerate they lose fluid and become dehydrated. Instead of a disc being well filled with a pulpy fluid gel – the nucleus pulposus – that supports and fills the space between successive vertebrae, you now find that two vertebrae may appear on x-ray to be closer together. Being closer together means that the ligaments joining one vertebra to the next are now slack, and are no longer able to stabilise that segment. While the muscles are in control, as in walking, all is fine but any static positions – standing, sitting or lying – are potentially a problem. One of the commonest activities to show this effect is 'stop start' walking, typically shopping. The standing around in a shop waiting at a counter or at a check-out producing the typical intolerable tiring ache in the back, as the muscles relax and the ligaments are forced to take the strain of the unstable segments.

Lying at night in a soft bed, for example, your 'flat tyre disc' can allow one vertebra to shear relative to the one below. The ligaments are then put under strain as they work to prevent you shearing any further. You frequently wake in the early morning, long before you wish, and then cannot get back to sleep because of aching from the overstretched ligaments.

First thing in the morning it's difficult to get out of bed, as you have to effectively stack one vertebra on another to assume an upright position. This is when you have to put your hands on your thighs, to push yourself up from a sitting position on the edge of the bed. This allows the muscles along the spine, the erector spinae muscles, to reassemble one vertebra on top of another.

At first, you probably can't straighten up fully. The computer programme is running but the components it's operating are not responding. Gradually your muscles are able to resume the control of your unstable segment, and you are able to straighten up. As you can imagine, until you have had a chance to establish this balance you are vulnerable. Amazingly, once you are upright, with the vertebra-flat tyre-vertebra arrangement under control you may feel quite normal. It's the movement from a static position, sitting or lying, that highlights that there is a problem.

## WHAT CAN YOU DO ABOUT IT?

- Sitting upright, with a cushion in the small of the back so that you protect the unstable ligament is essential. This particularly applies to long plane journeys.
- Having a bed with a good supportive mattress is another must. If the bed is too hard, it won't mould to support you. If it's too soft it allows you to sink too far and that's even worse. Invest wisely – you'll spend roughly a third of your life in bed! If your back is comfortable at night it will be better during the day.

### 'Waiting for the kettle to boil' exercises

Just as an athlete needs to train every day to keep his machinery in perfect working order, so we need to train our structures every day to keep them at their optimum functioning level. You really are only as good as today's efforts, so keep up with the exercises. We are so sedentary in our everyday life that they become essential.

- Practise the 'two orifices' exercise (see pages 102–3). You must keep working away at this one, it is so easy to do and so important.
- Walk, walk, walk.
- Balance on one leg.

Further help

Your doctor or an othopaedic consultant may refer you for an x-ray or MRI scan.

X-rays don't show discs, as they don't have calcium in them. They only reveal the vertebrae. If two vertebrae appear to be closer to each other than is normal, this indicates that there is a flat tyre disc between them. This is probably the single most common finding on x-ray. It is found just as frequently, on a routine x-ray, with people who don't have a history of back pain. Remember, x-rays are static pictures of a moving object; as such they can't actually tell you what's wrong.

If I were a clock repairer and took a photograph of your clock, from that photograph I would not be able to say whether your clock is going, has been going or will go tomorrow. I can have no idea if it is fast, slow or just needs adjusting. It is a static picture of a moving object and can give no realistic information as to how it works. Always remember that about x-ray and scans. They do provide information but they don't definitively tell you what's really wrong.

It's not the flat tyre, or loss of disc space, that gives you the pain, it's the ligaments coping with that situation, and the resultant muscular chaos, or loss of control, that determines the symptoms. You can't see this on an x-ray. So don't let yourself be fobbed off with, 'There, that's the cause of the symptoms, you will have to learn to live with it!' For when the symptoms have gone, the x-rays will still look the same. Providing you have an efficient ligament→nerve→computer→nerve→muscle feedback loop then you may never have back pain again, but your x-rays will still show the flat tyre and loss of disc space.

An MRI scan gives more information than an x-ray, but what

it can't do is to actually say whether it's hurting or not! You could have five people with varying degrees of symptoms, from nothing to severe, and, short of chance, you could not match the patient to the picture. The MRI scan showing the most minimal changes might be of the patient with the worst symptoms. Conversely, the worst picture might be of the patient who has never had a bad back in his life! So these scans must always be taken in context: clinical presentation *and* MRI finding.

An orthopaedic specialist may recommend some physiotherapy or other complementary medicine approach, but other than prescribing analgesics and anti-inflammatories will be unlikely to do anything else. At the end of the day it's down to you to look after yourself.

## WWW.ACUTE BACK PAIN

### WHAT IS IT?

This is the sudden crippling bout of acute immobilising back pain. Usually, but not always, there is a history of back pain, and now it can often be triggered by just a trivial reason – bending to pick up soap in the shower, or tying a shoelace – there is a sudden acute back pain and you are locked in a spasm, unable to move. When it happens it is very painful and very frightening, so let me try to take the fear element out of it by letting you understand what's happened.

WHY IS IT?

Almost certainly underlying the problem is some existing disc instability – a flat tyre. The movements that we use to operate the structures of the spine, through the feedback loops, are flexion, extension, side-bending and rotation. With these we can perform and control all our operations. However, we are neither able to initiate nor control shear.

Imagine now our flat tyre disc, which, like a flat tyre on a car, can shear the tyre wall of the disc. We make a rather casual movement to pick up a pencil from the floor. We are not consciously thinking of protecting our spine as it has not given us any cause to anticipate what is about to happen. Suddenly, at that unstable level, one vertebra slightly shears across the one below and sets off an explosion!

The ligaments around that disc are not programmed for shear, and so nerve signals rush up to the central control centre in the brain, which registers the computers equivalent of 'You have performed an illegal operation and will be shut down.' Your central nervous system, the brain, and its body control centre fire signals to the muscles around that segment, with all the components that it can muster – flexion, extension, side-bending and rotation. There is chaos. You are locked in chaotic muscle spasm, and no longer can you consciously order the structures to perform. No wonder it hurts.

WHAT CAN YOU DO ABOUT IT?

As with the earlier problems, the more efficient your 'loop', the less likely this is to happen. It's like the ballet dancer, with the sprained ankle and the wobble board. She needs to train the loop

THE LOWER BACK   111

to rehabilitate and prevent the problem from happening again. You could try taking more care when doing the actions that made this happen. The trouble is it's like biting your tongue; if you knew in advance it was going to happen then you could avoid it. The trouble is because normally it works so well, we take it all for granted.

### Immediate response.

How incapacitated you are will depend upon how many muscle components have been activated. At the worst all you can do is to lie where you are. Try to get on your hands and knees. This can sometimes work and, with the spine in its 'original' horizontal position, you may be able to move around. Trying to move will usually help.

Remember, you're trying to override chaos with order. Simple movements will start to help replace the chaos that has been created, with order. If you can manage to stand it will be a great help, though, as before, you may need to put your hands on your thighs to push yourself up into a standing position. If you can manage to walk a little, then running 'walk mode' as an old-established programme in your 'loops' will help to organise your chaotic muscle spasm and help restore control.

- If, at first, the pain is very bad, lie down and have some bed rest. Though the floor is firmer, if you have a firm bed or sofa available, you will be better off as it's not as difficult to get up from the level of a bed as it is from the floor. Lying on your side with the knees bent up in a foetal position usually works best.

- If you wish, take some anti-imflammatories, such as ibuprofen, as this will help reduce the pain and inflammation, and, if it helps you to be able to move a little, then it's worthwhile.

■ If you are really unable to move then a couple of days' bed rest will help the chaos to resolve, and gradual movement will restore order.

■ An ice-pack placed over the area for about ten minutes can help in the initial stages when the symptoms are very acute. Just as a sprained ankle swells as a response to injury, there will be swelling deep inside – you may not be able to see it, but assume it's there and treat it accordingly.

'Waiting for the kettle to boil' exercises
The 'two orifices' exercise will help to re-establish the control pathways again. Your whole system has been shocked by the event; you need to assure your system that everything is under control by exercising your authority. You'll amaze yourself at how quickly this starts to work.

Homecare
You certainly don't want to spend too long in bed. You might find, as you begin to improve, that lying on your back and pulling your knees up to your chest a few times will help.

When you can stand try, with your arms straight, to lean against a mantelpiece or the back of a chair, so that you can let your back gently bend, just a little, into extension. (See illustration overleaf.) Very gently! Everything is aimed at restoring order.

Further help
Your doctor may give you an injection of an antispasmodic, which can dramatically relieve the muscle spasm, although it doesn't

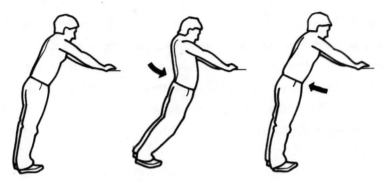

Standing Lumbar Extension

work for all cases. He or she will almost certainly prescribe a mixture of analgesics, anti-inflammatories and muscle relaxants. You may also be sent for an x-ray. But as I said earlier, there is nothing whatsoever on an x-ray – or an MRI scan – that will indicate that you have had an incident, are having an incident, or will have an incident in the future. What you will see is that you have a potentially unstable disc; but that's all. X-rays and scans are important investigative tools, when they are used to either eliminate serious pathology, such as fractures or tumours, or to identify nerve root pressures that will require surgical intervention, but they are of very little constructive value in the diagnosis of the vast majority of uncomplicated back pains. In many cases they may even confuse the issue, in that they may demonstrate some underlying degenerative state that is not primarily the direct cause of the symptoms. However, used in conjunction with a good clinical examination and case history, they can help in reaching a good assessment of any problem present.

Complementary medicine

Physiotherapy, chiropractic, osteopathy, acupuncture and reflexology can all help restore order. Remember, the problem often looks much worse than it is, and if you appear to be bending over to one side in a grotesque way, that's merely the unstable disc level with asymmetrical muscle guarding. You will not be stuck like that for ever. Just be careful and patient, and it *will* get better. Take it as a warning to improve your control loops, your neuromuscular integrity, and to be more actively in charge of yourself.

## WWW.ACUTE BACK PAIN AND SCIATICA/TRAPPED NERVE

### WHAT IS IT?

We now know all about back pain. This added complication is created by pressure on a nerve, in this case pressure on one of the components of the group of nerves that collectively form the sciatic nerve. The sciatic nerves runs from the backside, down the back of the thigh and lower leg to the foot.

It's important to realise that sciatica is not in itself a disease; it is merely a symptom of a fault. The trouble is that, because it is such a common symptom, we are all inclined to say, 'I've got sciatica' rather than look for what fault has in fact caused it. Most of the time, the fault is some factor of a particular disc.

### WHY IS IT?

At each segment of the spine – vertebra-disc-vertebra – a pair of nerves emerge, one from each side. To exit the spine, each nerve has to run along the back and to one side of the disc. This position is called postero-laterally, literally meaning 'from behind and one side'. If the disc bulges postero-laterally, it can pinch the nerve and cause severe pain. The nerve involved depends on which level of disc is affected. Because the base of the spine, whether we are standing or sitting, carries all the weight of the body, it's very common to find that one, or both, of the bottom two discs at the base of the spine becomes progressively squashed under the load. It effectively becomes like a flat tyre on a car. So this involves, either or both, the L4/5 or L5 sacrum discs.

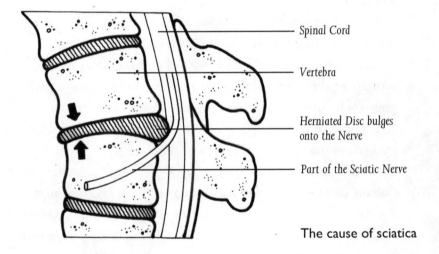

Spinal Cord

Vertebra

Herniated Disc bulges onto the Nerve

Part of the Sciatic Nerve

**The cause of sciatica**

The nerves from these two segments are part of the components that make up the sciatic nerve, the nerve that emerges in the back of the backside, to travel down the back of the thigh, lower leg and into the foot and toes. Slight pressure on this nerve can cause tingling, or a pins and needles sensation, usually at the end of the nerve in the foot and toes. It has the same effect as touching that nerve behind the elbow – the funny bone – and getting tingling in your fingers.

More pressure can lead to pain all along or in part of the pathway of the nerve. Even more pressure can lead to numbness in the pathway. That's really what sciatica is, a pressure on the sciatic nerve from a bulging disc. It can come on gradually or suddenly from a particular movement. The symptoms can be very severe as the nerve is about the thickness of a ballpoint pen refill. Think of the pain you get with toothache – that nerve is only the thickness of a strand of hair. Compare it with a nerve as thick as a ballpoint pen refill and you can understand why sciatica hurts so much.

Years of repeated lifting compress, and gradually weaken, the disc wall, so that one day, like the straw that broke the camel's back, it may be merely a trivial action that precipitates disaster. It is often bending forward to clean your teeth in the morning, with your back potentially vulnerable from lying flat overnight and your muscular protection not yet fully engaged, that is the simple movement that causes your sudden 'puncture'.

What happens is that as you bend forwards, your flat tyre bulging disc is squashed in the front, making its gel core bulge to the back. This causes the outer casing to bulge backwards suddenly, as with a puncture, forming a bubble of gel which presses against the nerve. As the neck of the bubble is narrower than the bubble itself, the gel is trapped and can't suck back in. This is a hernia, a bulging out, and is called a herniated disc.

The disc may rupture, the outer casing bursts open and the gel protrudes. This is then called a prolapsed disc.

It depends on whether the disc is actually pressing on the nerve root as to whether you get sciatica or just acute back pain. The nerve root has a sleeve around it to allow it to slide freely in its canal and as the pressure builds up on the nerve root this sleeve can become inflamed. When something gets inflamed it swells up, as with the blister on the heel with a too-tight shoe. It is also sore and it is the inflammation of the nerve root sleeve that causes the pain. If the actual nerve roots swells, the limited space it occupies means there is even more pressure on it from the bulging (flat tyre) disc. That *really* makes it hurt.

## WHAT CAN YOU DO ABOUT IT?

Usually, if the inflammation is not too severe, then lying down to take the weight off the disc, thus reducing the amount of bulge, will relieve the pain. If the nerve itself becomes inflamed, even lying flat in bed will be painful, and finding any position of comfort is difficult.

- Take to your bed and find the most comfortable horizontal position possible. This will probably be lying on one side with the painful leg uppermost.
- Try bringing one knee up in the foetal position, but keep the upper (painful) leg straight. This can sometimes help relieve the pressure on a nerve from the protruding disc.
- Or, still in the foetal position, draw yourself to the edge of the bed, and let both legs rest over the side. This helps to take pressure off the nerve root.
- You can also try lying flat on your back with the knees bent, feet flat, to allow a maximum degree of relaxation.
- You may also want to take an anti-inflammatory such as ibuprofen to reduce the swelling.

### Further help

Your doctor may suggest bed rest, analgesics, muscle relaxants and anti-inflammatories. This is to buy time to allow this acute situation to settle down. The disc bulge, like a tiny grape, will, in time, shrivel to a raisin and hopefully take the pressure away from the nerve root.

One of the most frequent common factors, that I find with my patients, is the appearance of a relative short leg on the opposite side to the sciatic pain. When you stand, you carry more weight on the short side, therefore you will bulge the disc to the opposite side. Making this symmetrical allows the body to balance centrally and this helps to reduce the postero-lateral bulging.

### Complementary medicine

An acupuncturist, physiotherapist, osteopath or chiropractor may help to relieve the symptoms and allow the condition to resolve.

### Surgery

An orthopaedic surgeon or neurosurgeon will certainly arrange for an MRI scan. Sometimes the scan will show such a massive pressure on the nerve root, and there may be such severe pain or numbness and loss of control of musculature in the affected leg, that surgery is essential.

### Epidural steroid injection

This is used as a halfway stage before surgery. Because the pressure of the bulging disc has inflamed the nerve and caused swelling in a confined space, if you can relieve that swelling, the symptoms can abate. This will allow time for the natural process of repair and for the disc bulge to reduce and shrivel, like a grape becoming a raisin.

Although this is done as an attempt to try and avoid surgery, if the disc is too protruded, then surgery can be a necessity. When it's all over you really need to take measures to protect your back against a relapse. The fact that one disc was a disaster can mean others aren't too hot either. It's like a tyre manufacturer recalling a tyre that might have come from a poor compound of rubber and can be punctured too easily. Our 'poor compound' may be a congenital weakness of disc structure, or just the fact that we overload the base of the spine in a very inconsiderate way. Only after the event has happened are we filled with sufficient remorse and desire to protect our vulnerable discs. Alas it's too late after the event.

All that I have described relates to our problems that arise through having a structure evolved and designed for horizontal use but one that we have used vertically. It is part of the high price we all have to pay for the benefits of sitting and standing upright.

# 8 THE MIDDLE BACK

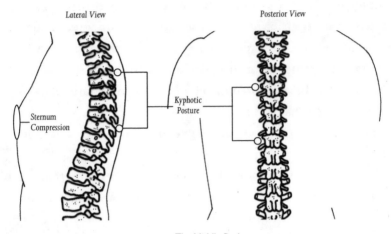

Lateral View                          Posterior View

Sternum
Compression

Kyphotic
Posture

The Middle Back

In comparison with the upper and lower back, not a lot actually goes wrong with the middle, though ironically it's the middle that is largely responsible for the faults that arrive at either end.

As we have seen, the spine is divided into cervical, thoracic and lumbar regions. These roughly correspond to the divisions of upper, middle and lower back that I have used in describing the problems that arise.

The thoracic (middle) section is the longest in the spine and is constructed out of 12 vertebrae and 12 pairs of ribs, to form the whole of the chest. It provides a safe housing for the two most essential organs in the body – the heart and lungs. The small but essential movements that the ribs make in breathing are necessary for the function of both heart and lungs. Allowing the thoracic spine to become too rigid, through bad posture, will therefore not only be a mechanical musculo-skeletal problem but also a physiological, functional handicap to life itself.

I am always delighted when patients comment on how they feel able to breathe more deeply and freely after treatment to help release a relatively rigid ribcage. They notice a sense of well-being at having been freed from restrictions that they hadn't really realised were there. When you live with a particular state for a long period of time it becomes your normal feeling and you don't realise that it can be changed.

## WWW.POSTURE PROBLEMS

Posture is always one of those words that seems to be an accusation. Oh, it's your posture!

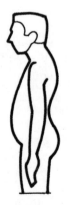 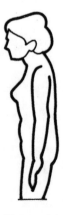 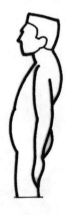

Kypho-lordotic       Too straight       Sway back

## WHAT IS IT?

Posture is merely our attempt to stand upright against the force of gravity. Posture is as individual as an individual. Certainly there is no single posture that is right and that everyone should adopt. Each must find the most efficient way to balance their body to give the best functional use of the spine. Too vertical and you lose the resilience that slight curves in the spine can give. You would find your teeth shuddering at every step you took from the jarring that transmits through a non-buckling spine.

If, on the other hand, the curves in the spine become excessive, then as the back curves out in the middle, the upper and lower ends curve in too much to compensate. That's when you get the ligamentous back pain I have described.

## WHY IS IT?

The middle back, or thoracic spine, with its 12 vertebrae is balanced with 12 more vertebrae, seven in the neck and five in the lumbar (lower back) region. What usually happens is that years of sitting badly makes the back bow out backwards. The muscles along the middle back (thoracic spine) have to fight against any weight in front. So, for instance, sitting with your arms in front of you, bashing away on a keyboard, requires a constant muscular contraction at the back to stop you keeling over on the desk.

Over a period of time, these muscles, often spanning several vertebrae, effectively splint the back into a rigid unit. You then get a back that is bent over forwards in the middle with several segments splinted together as a result of accumulated muscular contraction.

Now in very simple sense, if you have a back with some 24 or 25 moveable segments and you have six or so incapable of movement, you can easily see how this puts a greater strain on the others to make up for this loss of action. You end up with a rigid middle back brought about by enforced postural habits that compromise the function of either end.

## WHAT CAN YOU DO ABOUT IT?

You have to try and stop your children from developing the 'desk-sitter's' posture, described in chapter 4, as they grow up. Try to encourage them to sit upright at a desk and when eating at the table. I know what you're thinking, and realise it's much easier to say that than to actually achieve it.

During their teens they can easily change their posture habits, but, once into adulthood, when the structures are formed, change is much more difficult, if not impossible. As an adult, you can make you sure you have desks, chairs and computers at the right height. Bitch, moan, cajole, persuade – do everything you can possibly think of – to make your boss at the office give you a better workstation. You will never quite achieve perfection but it's worth the effort to make it as good as possible so that you don't become a victim of your environment.

'Waiting for the kettle to boil' exercise

■ Stand up frequently from sitting, clasp your hands comfortably behind your back, and try to make your shoulders meet at the back. Repeat a few times to stretch out the front of the chest.

■ Put your hands behind your back, push your thumbs in at

bra-strap level to make your spine curve backwards over your thumb. Do that a few times, then keeping the thumbs at that level, just push inwards a fraction, so that you are aware of that area, and of trying to flatten your back there. Don't try to pull the shoulders back. Just make your back straighten out a little at that point, and the shoulders will come back of their own accord. You only need a fraction of movement inwards to see how your shoulders automatically come back and drop down. To really feel it work, exaggerate the bad position and then correct it with the good one.

This simple exercise, done as an ongoing habit, is the simplest key to the best, most efficient posture.

### Deep breathing

Deep breathing, as a specific exercise, is something we all need to practise as most of the time we breathe in a rather shallow way. There are a couple of simple moves that can have a big effect.

- Stand up and place your hands on the top of your head with the fingers gently interlocked. Comfortably place the legs apart and then slowly bend to one side. Repeat to the other side, and continue alternating sides. Try to do this slowly and, at the end of each movement, accentuate the side bend to feel a stretch in the opposite arm. This really helps to open up the side of your ribcage, creating a space between each successive rib. It feels really good to do.
- Now do a few deep-breathing exercises. Stand comfortably, with the legs apart, take a deliberate deep breath in and, at the same time, stretch your arms up as high as you can. This

will help to open the lungs as fully as possible. Hold in the position for just a few seconds, to be aware of the feeling of stretch, then bend forward and let the arms drop down to try to touch your toes, while you breathe out as hard as you can manage. Try to make the out breath twice as long as the in breath. Just breathe out until you feel you can't wait to take the next breath. Try to repeat the cycle 10 times. Done each morning, this simple two-minute routine will help to de-programme the inactivity during the night and also, more importantly, help you start off the day without the typical compression at the front of the chest when sitting at your desk.

## Homecare

It's worth getting one of those Swiss exercise balls that you can lie against, and arch your back over backwards. Alternatively, roll a towel into a cylinder shape, and lie on your back with the towel placed under your spine at its most outward curve to act as a pivot point. Lie flat, with knees bent and feet flat so that your lumbar

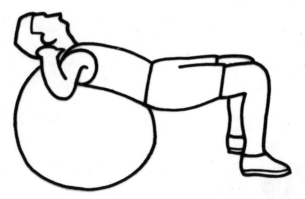

The back arching over exercise ball

spine is flat, and have a thin pillow or a book as a support for your head. Do this for half an hour every evening, and it will gradually help to counteract the effects of the daily hunching over the desk. As you do this you could listen to music, talk to the family or just relax.

### Complementary medicine

The various manipulative professions – physiotherapy, chiropractic and osteopathy – can all offer some help in getting that rigid middle to move a little. It would certainly be worthwhile to get some help and advice as to how much change you could expect. This will depend on the rigidity of the area and how long it has been established.

# 9 A DAY IN THE BACK OF . . .

Our whole life, from the moment of our conception to that of our demise, is about surviving evolution. Because, in many ways, we have transcended the evolutionary pathway of the common herd, we are especially vulnerable to the evolution that our intelligence as a species has unfolded. At the moment we sit on the wall, as it were, astride these two paths. We have not yet reached the stage, with our scientific development, where we are totally in charge of our own destiny, but are still hindered by the slowness of structural evolution to support us in this modern setting of our own creation. In this state we are simply surviving evolution, in a way that no other animal on the planet has ever had to do before. So this section is really about strategies for helping to deal with the situation.

Until we can find some way that we can genetically adapt our structure and function to allow us to be the master of our environment, we must make the most of what we have. What we humans have acquired, in comparison to other animals, is a relatively over-developed intelligence with a markedly underdeveloped musculo-skeletal system that is the root cause of most of our back problems.

In our busy, pressured world, few of us are willing to take the time and effort to make up for the loss of normal muscle tone that our very sedentary lifestyle has caused. We know we are too weak but need a simple solution for survival.

Without taking time out, but by just using those 'waiting for the kettle to boil' moments that inevitably arise in the course of each day, you can find solutions to your problems, and this is where I can help. For it to work, all you have to do in return is follow the suggested programme.

## SURVIVAL STRATEGIES

Earlier in the book I described the potential for the human animal: what we might attain if we pursued a goal. I also asked you to look at the reality – of the way we survive from day to day. If we can recognise our magnificent musculo-skeletal masterpiece, some- what gone to seed, then we can do something about it.

The difficulty is that the world we have created – office, desk, computer, car and chairs – constantly drags us down, by failing to stimulate our own trained muscular state, our proprioceptive circuit. If we want to survive without being the victim of back pain, we have to take responsibility for our machinery. We have to impose a regime on the structure, in order to keep it at a comfortable operating level. We do not need the bulging muscles of a dedicated weightlifter: in fact, very much the opposite. We need a sleek, finely tuned model that responds, with alertness and control, to our commands.

Very few of us are dedicated enough to spend hours daily at a gym to hone into shape our failing framework. But we do need to make up for the failure of our everyday workplace to naturally provide us with balanced exercise. What we need is a pattern or habit that we can simply blend into our everyday events to provide us with the necessary toning.

I will show you how to use everyday events to your advantage, so that you can make your existing day provide the exercise you need, without putting in hours at the gym. I'm going to take you through a typical working day, step by step, to show you just how simple it is to make an enormous difference to your back's health,

Remember it is not about developing large muscles but good proprioception – awareness of your body's feedback loops or circuits. If they work well you will be actively alert and able to respond to your surroundings.

## ACTION FOR LIFE PLAN

See how many points you can score in a typical day's action plan. First thing in the morning is a dangerous time. Before you stand,

| Rise and shine | Action | Score |
|---|---|---|
| 6.30 a.m. Sleep was a little restless. You woke at 5 a.m. and tossed and turned for an hour or so, trying to get comfortable. Just when it seemed you had drifted into delicious sleep the alarm goes. | Turn onto your back, with knees bent. Do 10 repetitions of the pelvic floor exercise. | 10 points |

remember your body has been horizontal for seven hours. Ease it in slowly! Ideally, just contract and relax every inch of your body – starting from your toes and gradually working upwards. Try to get each bit under self-control before you start to stand

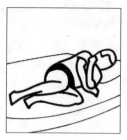

1. Lie on one side.
Hips and knees bent to 90° degrees

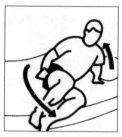

2. Push up with left arm and let
the weight of the legs help

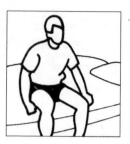

3. Sit still for a moment

**The safe and easy way to get out of bed**

## Getting out of bed

6.35 a.m. You should now be feeling a little bit more alive. Now is the time to get up. Getting out of bed is difficult if your back is bad, so always follow this routine. The correct movement, from the very first moment, when changing from horizontal to vertical is very important.

## Action

Turn onto your side – your left side if that is the side you will get up from. Bend your knees up to 90 degrees. Now, with the lower leg hanging over the side of the bed and keeping your body as one unit, push up with your left arm, letting the weight of your lower body 'pivot' you to a sitting position. Sit for a moment, but don't slump!

## Score

5 points

## Standing upright

Now stand upright, but think of how cats and dogs start the day – instinctively – and do the 'dog stretch'. This is rather like the stretch we often do when standing up. That arching backwards, arms

## Action

*The Dog Stretch*
This will only take two minutes from start to finish, so do make the time. Start on your hands and knees, with hands placed a little in front of your shoulders. Now, keeping your

## Score

10 points

pulled back behind you, and usually accompanied by a yawn. This the horizontal equivalent and much more effective. elbows locked, gently drop your upper body forward over your shoulders so that your back curves into full extension. Rest for a count of five in that position. Then smoothly lift your bottom and try to sit back on your heels. Rest there for a count of five seconds. Repeat this cycle 10 times.

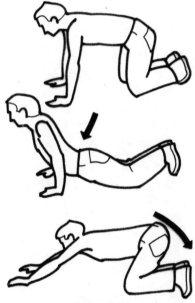

**'Dog' Stretch**
(Rest for a couple of seconds at the end
of each movement)

6.40 a.m. This is good. You have made it successfully into the upright position, are already feeling better and you should have scored 25 points!

## Shaving/Putting on make-up

Often, just standing first thing in the morning can be painful. Remember this is ligamentous back pain. It needs muscular control to support you. A perfect moment for a quick pelvic floor exercise. Note how you can't stand on one leg to do this exercise – you have to be balanced on both. It should feel as though your pelvic floor muscles are holding you round the pelvis like a wide belt. Instead of your upper body slumping into your pelvis to be supported by the ligaments of the pelvic floor, you are in muscular control. If you continue to practise this, over time you will completely change how you operate and control your posture.

## Action

*The Two Orifices*

As you stand try to squeeze your tummy against your spine. Also tighten the cheeks of your bottom, and 'hold' your bladder. It should feel as if you are lifting the whole of your pelvic floor. Hold it for as long as you can, then let go and relax for a few seconds. Repeat. Keep it going for as long as you are at the washbasin.

## Score

5 points

## Cleaning your teeth

A perfect moment for exercise.

## Action

Proprioception doesn't need muscle bulk – it needs balance. So come out of pelvic floor hold and do this little balance exercise. Simply stand balanced on one leg and then the other. Keep switching legs until you have finished cleaning your teeth. This is perfect for spinal balance.

## Score

5 points

So, instead of staggering out of bed in discomfort, you should have had a really good start to the day. Now for one more exercise, and that is the deep-breathing exercise. Because the daily confrontation with the office desk, or sitting in the car, produces compression in the front of the chest, and a closing up of the ribcage, it's necessary to start each day by de-programming yesterday's faults.

## Deep breathing

Stand comfortably, with legs apart, breathe in deeply and at the same time you raise your arms over your head, and hold the breath in for as long as comfortable. Then breathe out, while bending forward as far as you can, hold the position until you feel the absolute need to breathe in again. Repeat the cycle 10 times and award yourself 20 points for doing so.

## BREAKFAST

Have some wholemeal brown bread toast and some fruit – apple, banana, grapes. Try to feed your machine with loving care and control. You would not dream of stuffing a whole load of rubbish into the petrol tank of your car. Have the same respect for your body. Don't expect it to always just manage to extract what it needs from the junk you give it. Love your machine and it will give you good service for years to come.

## ON THE WAY TO WORK

The fittest I have ever felt was when I lived in north London and was able to walk to work, across Regent's Park, to Baker Street. It was just under two miles in distance and it took 30 minutes of fairly brisk walking. Walking is the single best return for investment. It is the perfect exercise for the lower spine and pelvis and a good exercise in proprioceptive awareness. It's also a great time for thinking, for getting those plans and ideas into shape. So take every opportunity to walk during the day.

| Getting to work | Action | Score |
|---|---|---|
| Standing in the queue or on the platform. | Do the 'two orifices' exercise (see pages 102–3). The more you do it, the longer you can 'hold' your pelvic floor. This will build up your muscle tone and give it that underlying state of alert readiness that will help prevent back injury. | 5 points |

| Sitting in your car | Action | Score |
|---|---|---|
| It seems so many people travel by their own transport. Sitting is one of the worst things that we do to our bodies. | Place a cushion in the small of your back to keep your back arched into extension. Most car seats are not good enough. Find the best and most comfortable one for you. You can buy lumbar supports from specialist shops, or use an old cushion, or small pillow – but do it! | 5 points |

## Stuck at traffic lights

A traffic jam is a perfect opportunity to add a few more points to the daily score.

## Action

You can do the 'two orifices' exercise (see pages 102–3) just as well sitting as standing. Try also a few shoulder shrugs, to let the upper back realise that it doesn't have to be round your ears! After shrugging, always try to let the shoulders rest in a relaxed position. Then, providing you keep an eye on the traffic, and only do this when you're stationary, let the weight of your head hang forward, so that you stretch the back of the neck, and then gently rotate the head from side to side a few times. Never waste a moment. It's only repeating the habit that establishes it.

## Score

5 points

## Travelling by tube/train/bus

Sit well back in your seat. Try to sit as upright as possible – don't slump. Always either walk to the next stop, or get off one stop early. Better still, walk the whole way if you can! Never let the journey be stressful. Use the time to be quiet and reflective.

## Action

Shrug your shoulders up and down. Let them drop. Tell them to 'relax'. Repeat 10 times.

## Score

5 points

### Walk to work

This is your best opportunity of the day to exercise and to build up your points score. If walking to work is not an option, try to find a 30-minute period in the day, such as during your lunch-hour, to take a brisk walk.

### Action

Time your walk and allow yourself one point per minute. A 30-minute brisk walk would be fantastic and give you a 30 points score.

### Score

1 point per minute

So, without actually materially altering your day, you should have so far managed to notch up 100 points or so for your fitness score. You have barely begun the day but you have made a constructive start. Don't stop there – the day is filled with self-help exercises for you to enjoy and bank. Think of putting points into your fitness bank account – each small deposit will be building towards your present and your future.

Let's assume that you are fairly office-bound and that, following a brisk walk (hopefully), you have just arrived at the office block. In the entrance hall there is a queue for the lift. What a wonderful opportunity to walk instead.

### Take the stairs

Try never to take the lift; instead walk up a few flights. If the whole journey is too much, take the lift and get off two floors earlier. If you managed two flights yesterday, try one more today. Don't forget to use the stairs to come down as well.

### Action

I said walking was the best, but probably stairs are even better. For each flight, one floor to the next, score 10 points

Going downstairs obviously does not require the same effort as raising your body against gravity, but it does require balance. So give yourself 5 points for each flight going down. So for two flights score 10 points.

### Score

Upstairs; 10 points per flight
Downstairs: 5 points per flight

## IN THE OFFICE

Sitting at the office desk is probably the single worst thing we do in our daily routine. We are simply not designed for prolonged sitting. In sitting the lower back takes the entire load, unsupported, of the rest of the body. Anyone with an acute low back problem will tell you the biggest difficulty they usually encounter is sitting. Around two-thirds of your whole body weight is compressing the discs at the base of the spine. There is no muscular support – it is only the ligaments that take the load, unless you take active steps to change this.

Listen to the office ergonomics advice teams. Get the right chair. You are going to be intimately related to your chair for a long while to come – try to make it a good marriage. For me, the kneeling chair is perfect, but admittedly I am always up and down from my chair.

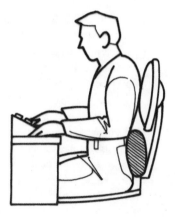

Good lumbar support
for sitting at your desk

If nothing else, I offer the same advice as for the car seat: find something – a cushion or lumbar roll – to support your back in the neutral position of slight extension, never slump in a backwards curve. This position, day after day, is a guaranteed recipe for disaster.

## SITTING AT THE DESK

Sitting at a desk is a game of halves: the upper half and the lower half. The lower half is all about compression from above. The upper half is about the postural habit and tension, of coping with the world that we have designed around us.

### Desk-bound

The problem is that it is too easy to get into bad habits. To start with you'll need to be aware of your body and its position.

### Action

At least every 30 minutes do 10 shoulder shrugs. Hold your shoulders up near your ears, then let them drop down. You can also roll them around – both backwards and forwards. Try to do this at least 15 times a day. Finish by really feeling the shoulders relax – let them drop.

Every hour, stand up, put your hands behind your back and try to make the shoulder blades meet at the back. Take a few deep breaths, in and out, before you sit down again.

Now let the chin drop forward to the throat. This stretches out the muscles at the back of the neck. Tension there leads to poor blood supply into the base of the brain and a feeling of tiredness.

### SCORE

2 points each time

## Mouse user's malady

We looked at this earlier and how the constant 'holding' tension leads to a repetitive strain injury and, if nothing else, tension in the muscles in the forearm.

## Action

Stop gripping the mouse so hard – let your arm relax, and find a support position for your forearm. Let go of the mouse and massage your forearm. Place the fingers of your left hand (if you are right-handed) over the muscles on the back of the right forearm, then roll the forearm, thumb rolling out to the right. This plucks the muscles and gets the blood supply back into them. Ideally, practise this at least every 30 minutes for one minute.

## Score

5 points per minute

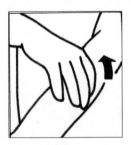

1. Feel Hard Extensor Muscles with your fingertips

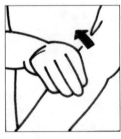

2. Start to roll the muscles towards you

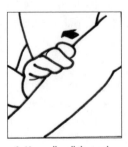

3. Now really pull the muscles towards you

Repeat the above movements about 10 times

**Forearm Massage**

### And so to lunch

Look at lunch-time as an opportunity to make up for your sedentary morning.

### Action

This is the perfect time to stretch the legs and add a few more points to your fitness bank by using the stairs and not the lift.

When you come back try to run up the stairs to get the pulse rate going a bit.

If time permits, add on a 20-minute walk in between.

### Score

Downstairs: 5 points per flight

Upstairs: 10 points per flight

You should be feeling pretty satisfied with your day so far. If you have done well and banked well over 100 points or so before lunch, then give yourself a pat on the back. You are already better prepared than before. Don't spoil it by having several pints of beer at lunch-time. Try to have some salad and something digestible – nothing too heavy.

### Back to the office

Another opportunity to put your body through its paces. Keep up the good work and be ever vigilant.

### Action

repeat the morning's exercises when you're at your desk.

10 shoulder shrugs
Make shoulder blades meet behind back, followed by neck stretch.
Massage forearm

### Score

2 points

2 points

5 points

| Time to stop work | Action | Score |
|---|---|---|
| There is nothing like a walk to get the circulation going in the legs. Or maybe you fancy a game of squash, football or tennis, or a workout at the gym. | Walk, walk, walk . . . See if you can muster up 30 points with half an hour's walk. You'll be surprised, if you're feeling tired it will actually refresh you. | 30 points |
|  | Game of squash, football tennis, or gym workout. | 50 points |

| On the journey home | Action | Score |
|---|---|---|
| Remember all the posture points and exercises from this morning's journey. Try to incorporate them in your journey home. They will help you recover from the stresses of the day. Do them when standing in the queue for the ticket office or bus, on the platform, on the bus/tube/train or when stuck at traffic lights. | 'Two Orifices' exercise. | 5 points |
|  | Shoulder shrugs followed by neck stretch. | 5 points per 10 shrugs |
|  | Head rotations/rolls. | 5 points |

## DINNER WITH THE FAMILY

You have done well. Time for some well-earned leisure. But that doesn't mean slumping in front of the TV. By all means enjoy your time for relaxation, but remember your back. Don't slump with your back flexed out, supporting your whole body weight. Sit as upright as you can and keep a cushion in the small of your back.

| And so to bed | Action | Score |
|---|---|---|
| When washing and cleaning your teeth remember this morning's balancing exercise. | Stand balanced on one leg. Change from leg to leg. You will quickly find that this gets easier. | 5 points |
| Before you go to bed, try a little stretching. | Do the Dog Stretch exercise that you did at the beginning of the day (see page 130). Try a cycle of 10 repetitions. This will help to get you in a relaxed muscular state before going to bed. | 10 points |
| When getting into bed, take care not to strain your back. | To lie down in bed, first sit on the edge of the bed and reverse the procedure for getting up. This will repevent any stress on your back. | 5 points |

If you have managed to notch up 250 points for the fitness bank on this first day then congratulate yourself, and try to repeat, or maybe improve on this tomorrow.

## GETTING TO SLEEP

Sleep, perchance to dream, or much more likely not to sleep at all, remains one of life's great mysteries and, sadly for some, an elusive commodity. For anyone with insomnia, those awful hours spent watching the clock tick by can be a real nightmare. Although we don't fully understand all of the functions that sleep fulfils, it is, without doubt, essential for our overall health, and it is a time for the body's repair mechanisms to weave their magic. Certainly all our musculo-skeletal dysfunctions can sometimes be made miraculously better after a good night's sleep.

I can recommend a couple of methods to help you switch to 'sleep mode'. This is where computers have an advantage over us. Once you have switched off all the programmes currently running, it takes just a couple of mouse clicks to put the machine into sleep mode. My methods may not be as quick and efficent but will usually produce good results.

## UNWINDING

The trick is to take your mind away from the day's stresses and put in calming control signals where you are the master of your thoughts and not the victim. If you are finding it difficult to get to sleep, lie back and, for a couple of minutes, think of times during the day when you could have found a few more moments of control.

Could you have done a few more of the 'Two Orifices' exercise? Perhaps a bit more shoulder shrugging? Walked a bit further, and more briskly? Tomorrow is another wonderful opportunity to use the environment around you as your personal gym and be your own 'personal trainer'.

### Muscular unwinding

This is an exercise in muscular control to make you the master of your function.

- Lying flat on your back, wriggle your toes and contract the muscles in your toes. Then let them relax.
- Contract the arch of your foot a couple of times. Then let it relax.
- Contract the calf muscles and then relax them.

■ Continue like this all the way up your body. Try to focus on as many areas as possible. Then, in turn, let them relax. The chances are that, by the time you have got to your shoulders, you will probably be asleep!

## Mental unwinding

If, by some chance, you are still awake, this is a pleasant game that you can play to drift into comfortable sleep. Having relaxed as many parts of the body as you can, it is now time to relax the mind. Uncontrolled, the mind can become distracted by a thousand trivia which seem important. The trick is to impose your favourite scene on it to overrule the unwanted images. For me it is to imagine playing a round of golf at my golf club, in north London. You can use your own scene of whatever makes you feel tranquil. The essence of it is to put as much detail into your picture as you can, so that you programme your system to override the unwanted signals that otherwise reverberate like a rubber ball in a squash court. Here's mine.

I try to imagine myself coming out of the clubhouse. I turn left, with the walls of the clubhouse on my left. There is a left turn around the side of the clubhouse and I can look across to the 18th green a few metres away and slightly below me. The scene across the 18th green is of the whole of north London.

The sun is slightly low to the left as I walk along to the first tee. I try to bring into memory every tree, every foot of the ground. I also, against reality, try to imagine hitting the perfect shot down the first fairway, then following it on to the springy turf towards the green. I think the furthest I have ever got was to the beginning of the third hole.

*

Try to find your favourite storyline and fill it with as much detail as possible. It is guaranteed to get you off to sleep successfully.

Remember good habits, like bad, are imposed by repetition. To get fitter requires a little effort. Each time you make these simple additions to your routine they become easier. So, every time you clean your teeth do the one-leg balancing routine. When you're waiting for a programme to load on your computer, do some pelvic floor exercises. Use every spare moment of the day to introduce new and healthier habits. This is the beginning of you being in charge of your own destiny. There is absolutely no doubt that if you introduce these good habits into your daily routine you will not only improve but also maintain your new health and fitness. The more established the habits become, the easier it all gets. Above all, make it fun – try to find more ingenious ways of scoring points for your health and fitness bank account.

It's like Pavlov's famous dogs that developed conditioned reflexes to salivate when a bell was rung and food presented. Once the routine was established they salivated at the sound of the bell even if the food was not there. If you keep repeating things until they become a conditioned reflex, you won't even know you are doing them. Each day, see how you can 'condition reflex' your body to become a finely honed machine. You can make your body a comfortable place to live in; it's up to you to put in the right input signals. Soon they will become your default setting, and a subliminal constructive part of your life that will better fit you to the world that you are in.

# 10 JUST FOR WOMEN

Women with their special structure and function are particularly vulnerable to back problems. For some the monthly menstrual cycle, with its changes in hormone levels, may in itself give rise to intense back pain. Similarly the structural and functional changes that occur during pregnancy, and the strains imposed lifting and carrying a baby in its early years of life, can demand a heavy toll on their body weakened by a sedentary lifestyle. Our ancestors, with their much hardier background, were naturally more prepared for motherhood than are the young mothers of today.

A look at some of the problems will help women to cope when the need arises.

## WWW.MENSTRUAL CRAMPS

Over the years I have seen many women who approached me directly concerning their painful menstrual cycle, and others who commented on the improvement in their menstrual problems while being treated for an existing back problem. There is one example that stays in my mind, as it was so dramatic.

I was working in India when a member of the staff there became bedridden with an acute bout of agonising premenstrual pain. I was asked to call to her room to see if I might be able to help. She was lying on her back in bed, knees drawn up. She looked pale and ill and was sweating with pain. She told me that this was a regular occurrence each month, but this occasion was particularly bad.

The way to treat acute conditions like this is to try and calm down the very marked chaotic spasm. So I put one hand under the base of her spine, the other over her lower abdomen. I could feel the waves of intense contraction and almost her pain. Slowly I gently suppressed each wave as it came against my hand. It's a subtle process that's like reeling in a fish on a line; you let the fish 'run' when it pulls hard and reel it in when you can. In a similar way, you have to let a powerful wave expand, and then suppress the gentler one that follows, until gradually the amplitude of the waves lessens and a feeling of calm remains. Gradually over the next 20 minutes the waves of spasm reduced until finally I could feel calm and order return. She gave a sigh of relief and I noticed that she had fallen asleep. I crept silently out of the room and whispered to her husband to let her sleep. The next morning I saw her husband at breakfast, and he told me that she had slept for a full 12 hours, and had woken up pain-free and well.

Over the last two years, since treating her, I have met her socially from to time, and she told me the problem has never returned to the same degree. Some months she is completely without pain, others she has some mild discomfort, but never as bad as previously. I tell this story because if one person can be relieved in that manner, it is possible that many others may benefit as well.

## WHAT IS IT?

Let me explain what I did and how it helped to relieve her symptoms. It always comes back to order and chaos. During most of our lifetime order prevails. Our bodies silently and simply carry out the most complex of functions, without our having the slightest awareness of their taking place. Occasionally, due to accident or fault of function, some factor upsets this grand order and relative chaos ensues. In the case of menstrual pain and spasm, the interplay of hormonal secretion and autonomic nervous system control that takes place in a monthly cycle just fails to harmonise. Blood vessels swell and engorge (fill to excess), muscles overreact and chaos replaces order. In this situation the body needs some assistance to recover. Damping down the waves of spasm provides the assistance for the body to regain control and allow order to return.

## WHY IS IT?

Sometimes there is a fault in how the sacrum, the triangular bone at the base of the spine, fits between the sides of the pelvis, at the sacroiliac joints. This may contribute to a disturbance of the autonomic nerve supply from the sacral plexus (a group of nerves that supplies many of the pelvic organs). In such a case, correction of the fault can improve the neural function.

In other situations, standing vertically, with the weight of the pelvic and abdominal organs bearing down into the pelvic floor, leads to congestion of the pelvic blood vessels, limiting the body's ability to function normally. In each case it's our upright posture that hampers the normal body mechanisms and prevents them from functioning in perfect order.

## WHAT CAN YOU DO ABOUT IT?

Fortunately, there are some useful ways in which you can help relieve the symptoms. Most problems in our bodies are merely functional faults, temporary glitches that in time will repair themselves. The more we understand the fault, and, more importantly, how body mechanisms function in repair, the more we can assist and speed up the process. Practical knowledge can be a very powerful tool.

Probably the principal problem in menstrual cramps is congestion of the pelvic blood supply and drainage mechanisms. Self-help treatment must look at how to assist the body to cope with engorged and painful blood vessels. There are two good simple measures that are worth trying.

### Ice-pack

■ Lie on your back, knees bent and feet flat, with an ice-pack on the tummy. In this position the tummy muscles are relaxed to help relieve the spasm. Putting an ice-pack on the tummy not only helps to numb the pain but it also reduces the swelling and increases venous drainage.

■ A packet of frozen peas from the deep-freeze is ideal for this purpose. Just wrap a thin towel around the packet and let it rest on your tummy for about half an hour. You can also buy specialised packs of a gel that can retain cold or heat. Keep one in the freezer and use it when necessary.

■ For simplicity, a cold wet towel, wrung out as much as possible, could be placed over the tummy and is very effective.

## Ice-pack with pillows

■ In more severe pain then try this slightly different approach. This time lie on your front with a few pillows under your tummy, so that your back is arched and your tummy supported by the pillows. This position allows the pelvic organs to hang as they would in a four-legged animal and takes out the compression and congestion from our vertical posture.

■ Now add the ice-pack treatment. You can put the pack on the pillows so that your tummy rests on it, or you can put the pack on the base of the spine, over the sacral area, the area that influences blood supply to the pelvic area.

■ You can also put a hot-water bottle under your tummy in this position. The contrast between the cold on your lower spine and the hot on the front can really stimulate the body's circulation. If you're really enthusiastic, try reversing the two – put the cold underneath and the hot on the spine. This can trigger the body's response mechanisms and help to restore normal function.

## Further help

Should you find that none of these approaches helps, consult your doctor to check that there are no underlying problems that need medical assistance. You may also find it worthwhile to consult an osteopath. He or she could check out your pelvic structures and make sure there are no problems affecting the pelvic organs or musculo-skeletal function.

## WWW.INFERTILITY

### WHAT IS IT?

Mostly, you don't know you are infertile until you try to get pregnant! Only after persistent attempts does the round of investigations start.

### WHY IS IT?

Congenital faults, previous infection of ovaries or Fallopian tubes, problems with male sperm, and psychological factors all play a part either together or individually.

### WHAT CAN YOU DO ABOUT IT?

Modern fertility clinics offer a phenomenal service to would-be parents – from implants to injections, so do consult a clinic. But for those who have tried all approaches and investigations and been told that there is nothing dramatically wrong that would prevent pregnancy, it is worth consulting a osteopath.

Osteopathy

You might wonder what osteopathy has to do with pregnancy. Well, osteopathy isn't just about musculo-skeletal structures, it's about making things in the body work properly. Every structure – be it ovary, Fallopian tube or uterus – has a structure and a function and can be subject to some degree of *dys*function. Sometimes – though not always – some simple osteopathic treatment can be the catalyst that helps restore normal physiological function to the organs of the pelvic floor.

I do some charity work in India and America for a particular organisation. When I was in India about two years ago I was asked to look at a couple who had been diligently trying to conceive for the previous six years without success. There was no obvious medical reason for their failure to conceive.

I saw the woman on three occasions and gave her treatment to the sacrum and lumbar spine, in order to influence nerve and blood supply to the pelvic floor and pelvic organs. I also directed treatment, using what we call the 'involuntary mechanism' (see chapter 13) to the organs of the pelvic floor, ovary, Fallopian tubes and uterus, particularly the pelvic fascia, to give support for the body's normal function.

Just over a year later I was in the United States, at the organisation's headquarters, where I look after newborn babies and children. To my surprise and great delight I was asked to see a three-month-old baby – a very healthy boy – who had been conceived within one month of my treatment on his mother in India! It was a very special moment for me to share with the delighted parents and their healthy son.

### Self-help

There are two exercises that may help to create a more receptive pelvic environment. Both help increase mobility in the lumbar spine and pelvis and help flatten the tummy. They also help place the cervix and uterus in a position that, if adopted during intercourse, will allow for better penetration. Practise them twice a day, in the morning and the evening.

■   Pulling the knees up to the chest

Lie flat on your back, and bend your knees and now clasp your hands round your knees, interlock the fingers and pull the knees as far as you can to your chest. Hold in that position for a count of five seconds, then let the arms straighten and return to the knees-bent relaxed position. Rest for three seconds and then repeat. Do 10 repetitions and then let the legs return to lying flat.

■ The pelvic tilt

You may already be familiar with this exercise, though it is sometimes difficult to focus attention to the right muscles. Lie flat on your back, knees bent comfortably and feet flat on the floor. Now, using the muscles of the lower tummy, tilt your pelvis. As you contract the lower abdominal muscles your bottom should lift just a fraction off the floor. Hold the contraction for a count of five and then relax for three counts. Try to do 10 repetitions.

Hot and cold compresses

If you are caught up in that dreadfully unromantic regime of measuring your temperature to judge when ovulation takes place, so that intercourse can be attempted at the most receptive time, then between telephoning your partner and him rushing home from work, there is something you might usefully do – and that's hot and cold towel packs. In the interests of romance, maybe do this before he arrives home . . .

All you need to do is have a couple of hand towels, one soaked in hot water and one in cold and wrung out until damp, then lie flat on your back, knees bent and feet flat on the floor. Put the hot towel on your lower abdomen and then alternate with the cold one. Just do 20 to 30 seconds of the hot, then the cold, for about 15 minutes.

Generally just learn to take care of your structures and understand how they work, as ultimately you are the only one that can.

## WWW.BACK PAIN IN PREGNANCY

### WHAT IS IT?

Some women say that pregnancy is one of the most rewarding periods in their life. For others it is a massive burden. Your body begins to change as the hormonal effects of pregnancy take hold. The mechanical effects of changing your centre of gravity can cause havoc. For so many women, having elected to delay pregnancy until later in life, comes the realisation that those years following a desk-bound career have left their mark.

### WHY IS IT?

The later in life you choose to reproduce, the more likely it is that the postural habits acquired through a sedentary lifestyle have become too well established. Sitting, very simply, makes you round-shouldered, weakens the abdominal muscles, and makes your lower back curve in, none of which is a great help in coping with the rigours of pregnancy. Remarkably, however, despite the extra load of the embryo, most women do fairly well, though when there is a problem it can be pretty severe.

The structures that take the biggest hammering are often the sacroiliac joints, and their ligaments. That's not surprising when you remember this is where the greatest changes took place when we evolved to the upright posture. Later in the nine months of incubation the sacroiliac ligaments soften to allow the pelvis to expand for the eventual birth. The mere mechanics of balancing the spine under these circumstances is pretty remarkable.

## WHAT CAN YOU DO ABOUT IT?

Women must take care not to lift too much. Remember, even a couple of bags of shopping will increase that load on the pelvis.

Try to get some rest lying flat on your back with the knees bent, feet on the floor. If the sacroiliac ligaments are sore this can give them a respite from the extra load that they are supporting.

This is a wonderful time in your life, with a remarkable event to enjoy, and if the enjoyment is not spoilt by pain so much the better. So do attend your antenatal classes, carry on your normal life but lift less, and rest when necessary.

Osteopathic treatment can help relieve the pains that come from the lumbar spine and pelvis, and I have treated patients up to the day before birth. Pregnancy doesn't preclude treatment, but it must always be carefully administered.

## WWW.MENOPAUSE

### WHAT IS IT?

Another one of those problems that women face and we men seem to escape. For some women they are unaware of it happening, for others it's a nightmare of different physical and emotional problems. I don't think it's normally a direct cause of back pain, but it can certainly aggravate an existing condition, and can cause real pain if serious loss of bone density (ostreoporosis) occurs.

WHY IS IT?

It's all down to a disturbance of the neuro-hormonal axis!

This phrase needs some explaining.

The evolutionary biological role of the woman is to bear children, and her hormonal chemistry is constructed for this purpose, the trouble is that sometimes, when the hormones that have been circulating silently for many years abruptly change, the body seems to lose the ability to resume normal service. We take ourselves so much for granted, never having to give a thought as to how internal systems balance our lives, that when some aspect of our internal household management system malfunctions we don't know how to cope.

An explanation about how it all works in normal circumstances may help in understanding the faults and how to deal with them.

The autonomic, or subconscious, nervous system is the one that controls our internal world against the outside one. It's our household control system. It controls our temperature, our digestion and our flow of blood supply. It controls saliva in the mouth, and secretion of digestive juices into the stomach. It controls blood pressure and the minute changes of blood supply to areas of the brain as different thought and action take place. It is your whole internal life support system.

At the same time the hormonal glands, pituitary, thyroid, pancreas, adrenals and, of importance in menopause, ovaries, sparingly ooze their secretions into the blood stream. The amounts of each are tiny; but then tiny changes can have large effects. The trouble is that many of the functions of the hormonal system mimic and augment the functions of the autonomic nervous system; hence the expression neoro-hormonal system;

the term neuro-hormonal axis refers to the balance of their interlinked functions.

A change in hormonal levels may well trigger a response in the autonomic nervous system that can result in a sudden inappropriate, and uncontrollable, rush of blood to the skin. A hot flush!

Bearing in mind the fact that the whole body could be affected, symptoms can vary from 'hot flushes' to digestive disturbances, profuse sweating, dry mouth, and also the well-known problems of bone density through disturbance in the way the body stores calcium in bone, resulting in osteoporosis.

It's all down to your biological clock deciding it's time to stop your reproduction mechanism and some of your other systems failing to cope adequately.

Back problems are not a direct result of these changes but existing problems may come to the fore with the changes in blood supply.

## WHAT CAN YOU DO ABOUT IT?

- First of all don't worry about it. The fear that everyone can see your profuse sweating is usually unfounded, your anxiety about it will only make it worse. Though for some it can last a long while, it is eventually going to settle down, and become one of those distant memories that one can barely recall.
- Fortunately we are in an era that has good medication for this situation. Your own GP may well decide to put you on hormone replacement therapy that will outwit your biological clock, and permit your body to continue to act as though you are still of child-bearing age. He may refer you to a gynaecologist who will monitor this treatment.

■ Bone density is a problem that affects us all, as we get older, but for women menopause may accelerate the loss of bone density and cause an increase in postural back pain. The vertebrae, particularly in the vulnerable thoracic area, soften and gradually change shape to produce that typical bowed-over thoracic kyphosis. You can prevent this by frequently doing the hands behind the back thoracic extension exercise. You can also try using a Swiss ball, and gently arch your back into extension. You can achieve the same by lying on your back and putting a pillow, or a rolled-up towel, as a wedge under the middle of your thoracic spine. It's usually more comfortable to have your knees bent and feet flat on the floor as this allows the middle of the back to relax over the wedge. Lie there for about 20 to 30 minutes each day, more if you can find the time. Done regularly this can be very effective.

■ Active exercising. One of the problems that faced astronauts, in the weightlessness of space flight, was the rapid deterioration in bone density (osteoporosis) due to lack of weight-bearing exercise. The level of calcium in bone is partly determined by the perceived need of the body to have strong bones. Use it or lose it is the maxim. The difficulty is that it is not just a matter of taking more clacium in the diet to restore levels, though dietary calcium helps; it is a complicated process involving hormone levels and active exercise. So, on advice from your doctor, take as much active weight-bearing exercise as you can, take supplementary calcium and also vitamin D that helps in the metabolic process.

# 11 JUST FOR MEN

Take heed you men out there. Our maleness is being rather too rapidly diminished. We are in decline and, at the present pace, we may soon be obsolete. Our contribution to procreation, though important, is a pretty poor show. Research shows that not only do we produce less sperm than our grandfathers, but what we produce is more sluggish.

## THE DESCENT OF MAN

In Steve Jones's book about the male chromosome, *Y: The Descent of Men*, he tells how the Y chromosome is being 'attacked' by the female chromosome, the X chromosome. We all start life as female until a set of genes turns some of us into males. In a sense we males are being feminised. A recent research project carried out in Scotland showed some quite extraordinary results. In a group of males studied over a period of 14 years there was shown to be a 29 per cent drop in sperm count!

### IT'S NOT OUR FAULT

Effluent from factories emptying into waterways and water tables contains levels of hormone-mimicking chemicals that have had a profound effect on nature. One study of coastal waterways showed an increase in female fish and a reduction in male. Similarly, among alligators in the Florida Keys there is evidence of a lessening male population with many males showing deformed male genitalia – sufficient deformity, in some cases, to prevent copulation. Take into account also the amount of female hormone being secreted into the water table from the vast amount of birth-control pills now in use, and our daily intake of feminising hormones is at a seriously high level. Apparently it is 'uneconomic' to filter out these hormones at water treatment plants so they pass, largely unchanged, into our drinking water.

Some bottled waters may have less hormonal contamination, or you could use a water filter on tap water. I am afraid that drinking beer instead is not the answer! Excessive alcohol can affect sperm levels, to say nothing of hampering performance; and, in any case, beer is made from water! So, if you want to make the best contribution to conceiving your child, probably the best you can do is be reasonably abstemious, not smoke and be as healthy as possible.

## PASSING THE BATON

Once that flurry of activity is over and several million sperm have hopefully launched themselves in the general direction of their target, the ovum, that's really all you can do for a while. So, for the next nine months, just be as helpful and supportive of your partner as you can. Meanwhile thank the forces of evolution that it is not your role to incubate the new, developing embryo.

## WWW.MACHO MALE MADNESS

WHAT IS IT?

It is the rush of blood that lets the macho male lift too much too often. The result being a serious low back injury.

WHY IS IT?

It is usually due to failing to realise his own limitations: not wanting to appear a wimp, and leaning across several people to pick a heavy suitcase from a carousel at a ridiculously wrong angle, or perhaps gardening for ten hours on a Sunday to finish everything in one day. No matter the event, the cause is an unrealistic view of his own ability given that a normal day is typically ten hours spent sitting at a desk in front of a computer.

WHAT CAN YOU DO ABOUT IT?

- You know the solution, just think before you lift!
- Place an ice-pack on the base of the spine for 20 minutes – always the best approach in an acute situation.
- Taking anti-inflammatory such as ibuprofen may help.
- Depending on the severity of the problem, seek help from your GP or complementary therapy.
- Just remember to be more careful next time.

# 12 SEX IN THE CITY

Sex, wherever it takes place, will always remain one of the most bizarre of all animal activities. The media, in every form – from newspapers and magazines, to books and films – devotes more time to its intimate aspects than to any other subject. It is apt that I should similarly devote some time to it. Just remember that there are always a few common pitfalls, and a few unusual ones, to take heed of. As always, prevention is best, and some knowledge of what can go wrong, and why, will hopefully help put you in charge of the situation.

## A TOUCH OF CLASS

If you've ever seen the seventies' film *A Touch of Class* you may remember the classic scene where George Segal is attempting a clandestine weekend in Marbella with Glenda Jackson. Just before the imagination of his physical desire can become a glorious reality, disaster strikes! A sudden muscular spasm in the muscles of the lower back renders him tragically immobile, and for certain incapable. It's a prime example of how, in someone with an existing history of recurrent episodic acute back pain, a trivial movement can trigger a painful attack. Sadly, even with the best back, things can go wrong at just the worst possible moment.

## THE MISSIONARY POSTION

George Segal's 'moment' was, if I remember, from getting undressed too eagerly. A far more common occurrence is for the man to be lying on top of his partner and taking his weight either on his hands or elbows. The problem is this position puts the lumbar spine into hyperextension – bending backwards too much. Add to this a few thrusts delicately, or even forcefully, forwards, and you have a potentially hazardous situation.

Some years ago a friend relayed to me his own unfortunate tale. Our young Lothario, to give him a pseudonym, had his first job working for a brewery in Burton-on-Trent. He had been dating one of the young secretaries at the office and at last had been invited back to her house while her father was on the late shift at the local colliery.

The house was in a small terrace, the tiny back garden led into a kitchen and, through a half stable door, to a very narrow parlour that housed a Rayburn coal-burning stove. Romance was blossoming, albeit in a somewhat cramped position, twixt a sofa and the Rayburn. Garments were being removed and he told me that there was a very pleasant glow felt from the fire on his now naked white backside. Picture now passions rising, time forgotten, with the soporific effects of the fire adding to the pleasure.

Suddenly Lothario was shocked by the sound of someone entering the kitchen from the back door. The next moment the upper half of the door was pushed open to reveal a black face, white-rimmed eyes and a Davy lamp on the forehead. Father and Lothario were locked, both in their own shock and horror, in a moment of frozen time.

Where, previously, the gentle rhythmic warmth of heat on

delicate white skin had been pleasant, Lothario now found that a prolonged moment in this position was becoming far too close for comfort. With a totally – I have no reason to doubt otherwise – involuntary movement, he was forced to give one thrust forward, impelled, he assures me, by the now intense heat threatening second-degree burns to the delicate skin of his behind. This action broke the deadlock. No words were spoken as father turned on his heel and strode back out of the house. Lothario, maybe cowardly but perhaps wisely, grabbed his clothes and ran for the front door.

## SEX AFTER SIXTY

Bearing in mind my own 65, or thereabouts, years on this planet I would like to look at some of the problems that may occur for some of my more mature readers.

Looking at males first, there is yet another glaring example of how our intellect has outpaced our physical animal and its inevitable decline with the passage of the years. The great male liberator, Viagra, may work wonders for the erectile function of the penis but alas does nothing for the erector muscles of the lumbar spine! Our intrepid male, suddenly being in the possession of a symbol of male pride, probably not seen in that form for many a year, can be led to attempt to perform with the rest of the machinery in a somewhat, let's say, cavalier manner. The frequent result of this is either the 'Touch of Class' syndrome or at least the stirring up of an old back pain the next morning.

As with any piece of complex machinery, the back is only as good as its weakest part. By 60, and usually many years before, the cumulative effects of standing and sitting have produced a fair share of problems in both the upper and lower back. Both of these areas will have been aggravated by the typical 'desk-sitter's' pattern of a fixed, bowed forward, middle back section. This in turn makes the neck and lower back curve into extension in the opposite direction as a counterbalance. Take the typical male missionary position – the hyperextended lumbar spine combined with the pelvic thrust forward motion – and you have the sound basis for flaring up an old back problem.

## THE FARNBOROUGH AIR SHOW SYNDROME

Meanwhile, the upper end of the back, where the base of the skull meets the top of the neck, is doing much the same thing, going into a hyperextension position. You are probably laying the foundations for a touch of Farnborough Air Show syndrome! What, you may well ask, is that?

Always after the Farnborough Air Show there was a glut of patients with stiff necks and vertigo. Standing looking up at the sky, to watch the aerobatics and presentations, with a vulnerable neck, the bending backwards of the base of the skull on the top of the neck, can irritate the complex mechanisms that control the blood supply to the base of the brain. Some people, if the position is held for too long, can faint, because of the loss of blood supply to the sensitive centres in the base of the brain. For others, the result of doing this for a prolonged period leads to an irritation in that critical sub-occipital area at the base of the skull, and affects the delicate interplay of the nerves and blood vessels that contribute to the balance mechanism.

Now, sadly, the Farnborough Air Show is no more, but there is always a steady influx of the 'sex after sixty' brigade, who present with a touch of vertigo and a stiff neck, following a little light entertainment that perhaps was a little more energetic, and slightly more prolonged, than usual. The similarity is, that in the horizontal face-down position, the male is forced to bend the head backwards, in much the same way as standing upright looking up at the sky. To those in this position all one can say is enjoy it while you can and may I suggest some remedies.

## A CHANGE OF ADDRESS

I don't mean that you should leave home; I am merely suggesting that you may consider a different position to face your loved one.

Try to adopt more of the side-lying position, with less of the 'macho' up-on-the-hands-and-elbows stuff. The latter might have worked 40 years ago, but if you want to play again tomorrow, a little sense and caution today is appropriate. Another approach is for the female to go on top. Certainly if it's the man who has the major back problem, then this will protect his back enormously.

It may depend of course on the weight of your partner and how enthusiastic she might be. It's all about communication and discussing each other's needs so that you can both enjoy a healthy sex life by avoiding painful situations. Experimenting to find the best positions can be fun and help to bring variety to your life.

## ARTHRITIC HIP

Enough of the male for the moment, let's have a look at the female. One of the first signs of an arthritic hip is a loss of what is called abduction. 'Adduction' and 'Abduction' are two words that describe movement. Adduction is bringing a leg, or an arm, for example, to the mid-line of the body. Think of it as bringing the legs or arms towards each other – you are *'add'*ing them together. Abduction is the opposite; it's taking them away from each other.

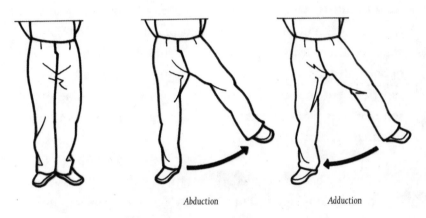

Abduction                    Adduction

An arthritic hip, therefore, can mean a woman no longer finds it easy to move her legs apart. At first it is barely noticeable, but as the wear and tear process of an arthritic hip makes itself felt, it not only restricts the movement, but any attempt to do so also becomes increasingly painful. This is a real turn-off for making love, especially if your man has found new vigour and enthusiasm, maybe as a result of taking Viagra, and is finding your somewhat less than enthusiastic response a bone of contention.

It is usually one leg that starts off the process, though it may well happen later in the other one. Let's imagine you begin to find it increasingly painful, and even impossible, to move the left leg to the side.

It might have come to your notice during, or after, love-making, when you have tried to open your thighs, that there is now a nasty pain in the groin on that left side. The weight of your partner has been inadvertently forcing open a reluctantly moving hip joint. The hips, flexed up a bit, are now being forced into 'abduction' – away from the body. For many women this is the first sign of an osteoarthritic hip joint.

At this early stage you are unlikely to need – or to be offered – a hip replacement, you just need some practical advice on how to cope with it. At least identifying the condition early gives you an opportunity not only to make some improvement to the joint function, but to help remove that element of pain that stops some of your pleasure. Here are a few suggestions that you may find helpful.

- If sex has been scheduled, or you think it may be likely, then trying taking some ibuprofen. By reducing inflammation, this may not only take away the pain but also improve the range of movement. You need to take it at least half an hour before the intended activity for it to be effective.

- Look at the hip exercises included in the exercise section starting on page 206. Certainly swinging the bad leg while standing on a couple of telephone directories will help. So too will lying on your back, knees bent, feet flat on the floor and then allowing the legs to fall away from each other as you breathe out. You almost have to 'will' the legs to gradually relax.

- If the pain persists and the condition is getting worse then you should consult your doctor who will probably arrange for you to see an orthopaedic consultant with a view to hip replacement surgery. For those who have had a successful hip replacement the relief can be enormous.

- Various other physical therapies can be very helpful before the need for surgery. Acupuncture, chiropractic, osteopathy and physiotherapy can all help to improve the condition, though if it is a genuine osteoarthritis, it is only a help, not a cure.

- Meanwhile, a little adaptive technique would be worth pursuing. Very simply it's the side-lying, or semi-side-lying, techniques that offer the simplest and best rewards. The simple side-lying approach, with your good leg flexed and the painful leg straight, not only provides great intimacy, but also solves the painful hip problem. If you can't get your left leg to open wide then just keep it straight!

- Sex on top can take away the pressure of your partner forcing an unwilling hip into abduction. Taking away this fear of the pain is often enough to allow you to relax and therefore permit more movement.

- When both hips have gone, I am afraid it is quite difficult to find a really comfortable position. At this stage surgery is probably the treatment of choice, but fortunately the hip operation is now an incredibly efficient procedure.

## RESUMING SEX AFTER PREGNANCY

During the latter stages of pregnancy, nature allows for the birth process by circulating a hormone that causes the ligaments joining the bones of the pelvis to soften and expand. Unfortunately, for some women the ligaments don't contract again as quickly and as well as needed. In that case the woman can be left with relatively unstable and over-stretchy sacroiliac ligaments after the birth.

Let's assume that you have decided to resume sexual relations.

This is the time to exercise great caution. By all means be loving, but also be firm, and don't give your partner the luxury of post-coital lying on top of you, which 'forces' apart your temporarily vulnerable sacroiliac joints. Stretching ligaments is quite difficult, getting them to shorten and stabilise is nigh on impossible.

Many are the times I have seen a very painful sacroiliac strain present under these simple circumstances. Once you develop an unstable joint like that, it does have a habit of repeating. Overstretched ligaments are extremely difficult to repair. Try not to let it happen in the first place. At least armed with relevant information you are in a position of some control. Use it wisely.

## STRENGTHENING THE PELVIC FLOOR

The pelvic floor takes a hammering during and after pregnancy, so it's important to make amends with the relevant exercises. Sucking in the pelvic floor will help enormously. Not only will it provide a stable base for the spine and pelvis but it will also help to tone the love-making muscles. Never waste an idle moment – keep repeating the pelvic floor exercise until it becomes ingrained. The uterus, cervix and vagina can be restored back to their pre-pregnancy state by really working at them. As well as helping you to reconstruct the vaginal wall, if you keep lifting the pelvic floor it will help you get back that flat tummy.

## OTHER SEX HAZARDS
Sex, with all its variations, will inevitably, in the heat of the moment, result in some unusual presentations. Here are just a few examples.

## JAW JOINT JAMMED

I once badly strained my jaw joint – the tempero-mandibular joint, or TMJ, as it's known in the trade. It must be 35 years ago, while I was on holiday in the South of France. I had, as it turned out a trifle ambitiously, tried to bite into a rather too large baguette roll. There was a sudden sharp pain in the jaw joint indicating that I had effectively 'sprained an ankle' in my TMJ. Over the next 10 days, rather than enjoy the lovely food, it was as much as I could do to open my mouth to push in an olive.

A few years ago a young woman consulted me with her jaw in a state rather reminiscent of my own experience. Her story was, however, slightly different to mine. She confessed, with admirable amusement, to a rather vigorous and enjoyable session of oral sex, and to have woken the next morning in this unfortunate state. Initially somewhat embarrassed to seek help, she had allowed the condition to carry on for several weeks before I saw her. Fortunately, after a couple of sessions of treatment to carefully rebalance the ligaments of the TMJ she was fine – and probably a little wiser.

There are a couple of useful remedies that you can do at home should the TMJ problem arise, be it from any cause.

### Massaging the ligaments of the TMJ

The tempero-mandibular joint can be felt just in front of the earhole. Opening and shutting the jaw, with the tips of your fingers over the joint, will give you the chance to feel it and do some gentle massage over the tender ligaments. Try using one of the anti-inflammatory gels such as Ibuleve, or a more heat-producing balm such as Tiger Balm. If you use the latter, take care not to get any Tiger Balm in your eyes, as it will be a real disaster.

Most TMJ problems will settle of their own accord in time, but you can usually speed up the process with a little gentle massage two or three times a day.

### Therapeutic jaw movements

You really need something like one of those rubber pencil erasers, about the thickness of your thumb. Place between your front teeth and gently bite, and at the same time try to slide the lower jaw under the upper one, so that you can feel the same sort of movement happening at the TMJ. This helps to mobilise the jaw joint and restore it back to normal function.

### Icing the TMJ

If the joint is really sore and tender then a little ice-pack treatment can be very effective. It's always a useful ploy in any acute strain condition. You really only need to do it for about 10 to 15 minutes at a time. After that, the therapeutic effect will diminish, but you can always repeat it again a little later.

## HEADACHE AFTER ORAL SEX

An old friend of mine came to see me with a most violent headache. When I questioned him more deeply as to how it had started, it transpired that he had been indulging in oral sex, with his neck and sub-occipital area in the Farnborough Air Show syndrome position. He had apparently been in this position for some considerable time. The result was that he had pinched that area under the base of the skull and had a real spasm in the muscles in the sub-occipital region. This is always a potential source of a headache.

ICE-PACK UNDER THE BASE OF THE SKULL

Once you begin to understand the body mechanisms in injury, the treatments become more obvious. If you know how something occurred, then a good ice-pack will work wonders especially if done straight away.

REVERSING THE INJURY

The problem arose from holding the neck in forced extension for too long therefore the best remedy is to try let the head hang forward, in the chin to chest position, so as to open up the area under the base of the skull. In this position you can try to gently roll the neck from side to side a few times to promote movement and relaxation of the sub-occipital musculature and improve the local blood supply.

AND FINALLY . . .

A chapter on sex should finish on a funny note; after all it is just about the funniest thing that the human animal indulges in. I still have great sympathy with one of my patients, who, learning about the birds and the bees at a rather late stage in her adolescence, indignantly and rather emphatically said, 'My mother would never have done that!' It is a fact that our mothers did do 'that' at least once in their lives, otherwise you wouldn't be around to read this today.

# 13 PROTECTING YOUR BACK FROM CHILDHOOD TO THE LATTER YEARS

The miracle of birth is for both parents to experience, the father should never miss this moment. Much of the previous nine months has been the domain of the mother, so it is now that the father can join in. But for now I am going to leave the parents aside, and concentrate on the journey for the baby.

## BIRTH

From now on, those two faithful twins, 'nature' and 'nurture', will interplay their roles to fully mould this new being into a unique individual. To fully understand these roles, I always think of planting a climbing rose. The colour, form, smell and texture of that rose are determined by nature, in its defining genes. How we look after it with water, food and support is the nurture we can give to help it achieve its full splendour. Nature has produced, through a unique set of genes, this individual, and now nurture can play a role in how we, as the parents, can help this child to realise its potential.

Your child has arrived at birth with some factory-loaded

settings to the hard drive. Life, or consciousness, has not only been pre-loaded but has been already running in the womb for several months. The new software programmes, of all future experience, may now be sequentially acquired. There is virtually no limit to the amount of programmes that can be loaded.

In this new 'outside the womb' world, our five senses – sight, sound, touch, smell and taste – are being sampled for the first time, giving us that rich experience of the environment around us. At this stage, each new input signal that enters the brain will help create a pathway of neural connection, that, once established, we will use to operate our structures and organs. This is the beginning of our formative years, when we grow in stature and knowledge, as we 'format' our systems for adult life.

## SYNAPTOGENESIS

A synapse is the junction point between one nerve and another, or the connection of a nerve to an end site, such as a muscle fibre or an organ. It's like a spark plug in a car, where an electrical charge jumps across a small gap, to thus complete a circuit. So, as we establish more synapses, we are able to build new circuits, of pathways and connections, so loading the software of reference and coordination. The process, of creating new synaptic connections, is called synaptogenesis. We can recognise objects that we have seen before and develop the coordination to use them. We begin to know what a spoon is for and, by repetitive use of a gradually established neural pathway, we can direct it to our mouth. That may be a simple task now, but watch your baby try to format the circuits that we have established on our hard-drives.

It would be practically impossible to overload this extra-ordinary biological miracle that is building itself to interface with the world around you. Sight, sound, touch, smell and taste, our senses, are essential to build up the brain's ability to experience the world. The more input the better. So expose your child, gently and lovingly, to all the experience that you can, so as to better fit him for his unique future journey.

## Objects to play with

Allow your child's manual dexterity to develop by letting them experience objects different shapes, colours and substances – the more the merrier. Remember always that at this early stage the mouth is the most developed sense organ, as it's first experience was suckling the breast. Be careful, as your child will try to initially experience everything through the mouth. So sharp objects and things that can be swallowed are out.

## CRAWLING

This is that time to relive our evolutionary past and exist in our world on all fours. There is practical evidence to show that proper crawling is a necessary process for integrating coordination. So encourage crawling, and certainly don't try to make your baby walk before he or she is good and ready. It doesn't matter if next door's child started walking at 10 months and yours is now 14 months or so! The longer the crawling, the more chance spinal and abdominal muscles have to integrate with the upper limbs, lower limbs and the spine. I'd always advise against those baby bouncers. There will be enough time standing for the rest of his or her life, so no need to rush it now.

## FIRST STEPS

This is always one of the most exciting milestones for parents to see. But if you make your child walk too quickly, without having built up the use of the spinal and abdominal muscles, you run the risk of their having postural problems for the rest of their life. The moment the baby stands he or she will start to load the software programme called 'WALK' that they will run – on demand – for the rest of their life. This is the beginning of that process of 'proprioception' that we looked at earlier.

The feedback loop of teaching the brain to listen to the input signals from the ligaments and then to command respective muscles to balance and walk is what is happening.

Each time your child falls, then gets up and gradually balances, the brain is learning and establishing the millions of loops necessary for enabling the child to walk and balance in the smooth way that we adults have now achieved, and take for granted. If the abdominal muscles have not been developed from crawling, then your baby will tend to stick its bum out, and its tummy out, in order to balance. You then have a very curved-in – hyperextended – lumbar spine, whose shape will be etched into the developing computer programme of balance.

If the baby learns to walk with this shape, he or she is more likely to remain that way, as those are the component loops that are being hard-wired into the system. Think about it, and stop worrying that your precious bundle is apparently two months behind next door's baby. Yours may be much better off in the long run.

## GROWING UP

We have the longest growing-up period of any animal on the planet, as we have the most adaptable brain that is just waiting to be loaded with all the software we can muster. Fortunately as far as our musculo-skeletal development goes, most of the first few years go pretty well. If you have any concerns about your child's posture, take them along to an osteopath or an Alexander therapist, who can help. Get competent professional advice first before you give your child any exercises. There is a charity clinic in London called the Osteopathic Centre for Children where children from birth – even in incubators in hospital – to about the age of 16 are seen. Parents are encouraged to bring in their newborns, from two or three weeks of age, for a check of their systems. These are the subtle systems of our developing function that help the baby achieve its full potential. It is well worthwhile, very gentle, and employs delicate cranial techniques that are particularly effective at this important early stage of growth. I know this because I have worked there and also had both of my children successfully treated there.

### CRANIAL OSTEOPATHY

Perhaps this is the moment to explain 'cranial osteopathy' (see also chapter 16) as this is relevant to your child's development. Though this is a relatively new concept, the structures, and with them their function, have been there since vertebrates first roamed this planet.

I remember, having just finished my first post-graduate course in cranial osteopathy, taking my daughter to the Natural History Museum and seeing there the skeletons of dinosaurs. There, in the skulls of these massive and unlikely-looking creatures, were the very structures that I had been handling in human form a few days earlier, and had marvelled at the intricacy of their form and action.

Until you have felt the involuntary motion of the body, and the particular way that the skull bones are involved in this perpetual rhythmic motion, it is virtually impossible to fully comprehend the profound importance this has in the body. That cranial, or involuntary, motion exists, I have absolutely no doubt. I have equally no doubt that it performs some necessary process in the body – it would simply not exist otherwise. Exactly what that function is, I accept, must remain open to some conjecture, so what follows is my hypothesis.

### The magician, the radar beam and the involuntary mechanism

You know those children's entertainers who make wonderful animals and shapes out of balloons? The magician manages to blow up a balloon and then with a bit of blowing, some pulling and pushing and certainly a lot of moulding of the balloon with the hands, is able to make all manner of shapes.

When a baby is born it's almost as malleable as the magician's balloon and our 'baby balloon' grows at a rapid rate. At the same time there is a rhythmic motion of contraction and expansion, repeated over a 10-second cycle, which osteopaths refer to as the involuntary mechanism. This rhythmic cycle can be felt any-where in the body – not just in the cranial (skull) bones.

The ongoing, genetically encoded intelligence is gradually building the baby from its master plan, and each rhythmic cycle is rather like a radar beam bouncing a wavelength against objects in its path and then imaging them on a screen. Likewise, our involuntary mechanism feeds back a 'picture' of our whole body. The magician 'knows' what he is going to build from the initial lifeless balloon that he stretched between his fingers. So, too, our 'intelligence magician' knows that it is going to form the baby balloon into a 5ft 8in tall, beautiful blonde lady with blue eyes and peach-coloured skin. Each sweep of our 10-second involuntary radar mechanism feeds back information as to the progress being made, like a builder checking that the construction is accurate according to the plans.

Now let's imagine that there has been a difficult birth, perhaps a little too long being pushed against a reluctantly dilated cervix, or maybe a torsion strain in the womb – the potential for minor forces to warp the balloon are many – that has been imposed on this young person. Time then to call for the 'intelligence magician's assistant', in the form of an osteopath adept in the use of the involuntary mechanism, to delicately mould the 'baby balloon' back to the maker's specification. This may be a fanciful way of looking at it, but in essence this is what can be done.

Earlier this afternoon a friend called by to show off her lovely five-month-old baby daughter. She told me that she had taken her daughter to a local osteopath, who had good paediatric experience, as her baby had shown a distinct side-shift of her upper body in relationship to the base. This was, she thought, the result of a fairly traumatic labour. Two treatments later, of gentle involuntary mechanism techniques, the problem had been completely remedied. This may not be 'self-help' but it is an invitation to help yourself by taking your baby for a check-up – even if there is apparently nothing wrong – so that the intelligence magician's assistant can assess that the 'baby balloon' is true.

As a practitioner you are able to pick up the subtle pressure variations in the baby balloon and recognise them as faults. At the early stages they literally just melt away in your hands, and you feel the tissues almost seem to give a sigh of relief as they are corrected. The longer a fault remains, the more established it will become in the system. It's as if the involuntary mechanism radar beam becomes used to the reflected pattern of abnormality, and it continues to build the balloon, accepting as normal the fault pattern. Don't let that happen. It is usually so easy to correct these faults in the first few months, and thus allow a perfect growth pattern to proceed normally.

## THE TEENAGE YEARS

It's often at this stage, as we progress towards maturity, that the postural habits conditioned by our environment become the established patterns for our adult life. Nature, following the instructions inscribed in our unique genetic code, is busily finishing its building process, but it is now, too, that nurture may play its part in securing our future shape. It's only by the understanding of nurture's role that we can hope to make our active contribution to the quality of the finished product. It really is a window of opportunity that must not be missed.

### WWW.FIRST BUST IN THE CLASS

#### What is it?

This is bending over forwards with rounded shoulders – in medical terminology, a thoracic kyphosis. It's not just the middle back or thoracic spine that is the concern, it's more about the curves in the neck and lumbar spine that have to compensate. We will see more of these when we come to the upper and lower back problems of adult life.

## Why is it?

This, sadly, is one of the most common problems for a young girl, and it is probably the single greatest factor for producing a lifelong postural problem that she is likely to experience. It need never be a problem if it is addressed properly at the outset.

It's caused by the social embarrassment of developing either the first, or the biggest, bust in the class. In order to avoid being the butt of jokes and attention of lustful male stares, she desperately attempts to hide her unwanted precocious development by curving forward in an effort to flatten the chest. Now, with the added influence of the inordinate amount of time spent posturing forward over a computer terminal, busily accessing chatrooms and sending emails, the problem is doubly compounded.

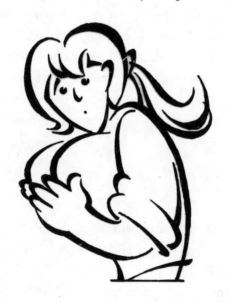

I can't tell you how many times I must have seen women in their mid-thirties having had their 1.8 or 2.4 children, and are now presenting with lower back or upper thoracic pain. Looking at them, and their presenting posture, I can often deduce that they had the first bust in the class at age 12 or 13.

### What can you do about it?

The first thing for parents is to be aware of the situation, and whatever you do, don't make jokes about it or take it lightly. This can be a real problem unless tackled with understanding and care. It's one of the 'nurture' situations of 'Postural Adaptation To Environment' (PATE) from standing and sitting upright against gravity. Fortunately, at this time in our pathway to adulthood, the spine is still malleable and can be adapted for good or bad, and there are some realistic measures to adopt that will make a difference for the future.

One of the best ways to help is to ask the young girl to imagine that she has sewn some barbed wire into the back of her bra strap. This means that if her back curves backwards she pushes against the wire and it will hurt, but if instead she pivots in at that point, then it's fine and it doesn't hurt. It's important to be aware of deliberately pivoting in at the middle of the back. You must not try to force the shoulders back, but just put a thumb at the point in the spine, roughly where the bra strap runs across, and then try to straighten up at that point. As the back comes out of flexion, and straightens up, so too the shoulders automatically stop rounding and will come back to their neutral position. If you do this properly you can immediately feel how it works.

Your input as a parent may be difficult to impose, whereas a physiotherapist, Alexander technician or osteopath can treat the problem and explain it in a way that is more acceptable for the young girl.

## WWW.TALL BOY IN THE CLASS

### What is it?
This is a bent-over-forward upper back, which leads to round shoulders.

### Why is it?
It's the boy's equivalent of 'first bust'. In this instance it's not the embarrassment of a developing bust but simply growing a lot taller than the rest of the class and peer group. In our teens none of us likes to be different, and, in this case, literally standing out from the crowd is the problem. So the tall boy stoops down to join the rest of his friends, setting in motion input signals that will give him a flexed thoracic spine, and curves above and below as a counterbalance. In doing so he is laying down the seeds of back problems that will plague him for the rest of his days.

This is further exacerbated by his environment, which was built for yesterday, and doesn't fit him today. It is no longer uncommon for the average class of 16-year-olds to be anything from 5ft 2in to 6ft 2in yet most are still sitting at the same height of desk! Through nutrition and evolution we have outgrown the modular scale on which our everyday furniture has been based. Ideally we should have desks that can be adjusted to fit the individual. At the moment the variable individual has to fit the fixed environment.

What can you do about it?

Encourage the use of a Swiss Ball. They're very good to sit on at the computer as they make you balance on them, and not slump. You can also use the ball as a back extension exercise gadget. All you need to do is lie with the middle of the thoracic spine against the ball, and allow the back to arch over it. This is likely to be more productive than constantly saying, 'Oh for God's sake, sit up properly!' Remember, the teenage years are the running-in period that determines the shape of the spine. The soft bones of the early teenage years become the hard bones of adulthood and will likely remain in that same shape for the rest of their lives.

## WWW.SPINAL OSTEOCHONDRITIS

What is it?

There is a specific developmental condition that is present in more than 10 per cent of the population. It emphasises existing postural problems even more by giving a postural pattern of thoracic kyphosis (bending forward with rounded shoulders), accompanied by excessive tiredness and aching in the middle and lower back, particularly after sport and at the end of the day.

Why is it?

The bones of the spine, the vertebrae, have comparatively soft surfaces which harden during our teens. It's the bones' equivalent of milk teeth, though, fortunately our milk bones don't fall out, they just mature.

In about 10 per cent of the population the process doesn't work too well and instead of going from milk bone to adult bone, there is a period of a few years when it goes to excessive milk bone. The reality of this is that the over-soft bone often gets shaped, and you are left with a thoracic kyphosis, a 'curved out' piece of back, that can become very stiff and totally set.

## What can you do about it?

The first thing is to recognise that there is a problem. Too often the symptoms are dismissed as 'growing pains'. But in this instance they are *real* 'growing pains' and need to be looked after carefully if the back is not to adopt a bad thoracic curve later on. If you have any concerns that your child may have a problem, do have it checked out by the doctor. You can then put in place the measures that will best help the remedial process during those important formative years.

- A Swiss ball as an exercise aid can be really worthwhile. You can encourage your offspring to do exercises leaning backwards over it to encourage the extension of the thoracic spine. As before, the Swiss ball can also double up as a seat to sit on at the inevitable computer desk. This can be effective in helping both posture and balance.
- Make particularly sure that the beds are really supportive, and that they don't sag too much. Soft beds not only cause the back to be very painful at night but will further exacerbate the hyperflexion in the thoracic region.
- Some help from physiotherapy, osteopathy and, in particular, Alexander technique will be an investment for the future.

General considerations.

As we become more and more sedentary in this modern world of ours, and our children become less physically active through hours spent with TV and computer, there is a commensurate rise in the incidence of back pain in children, so it's important to encourage more exercise. Make them walk more and ride less. Too often parents are guilty of driving children everywhere by car, for both convenience and fear of letting them out alone. If it is a question of a short journey that really doesn't need to be done by car, then walking with them will do you both good.

Have a look at the daily action plan in the earlier section (see page 129) and get them into the habit of amassing points for exercise. If they develop the habit young it could help to change their lives for ever.

## TOWARDS GOLDEN POND

To those of you who can immediately conjure up a picture of a dark lake, a rowing boat and blisters on the hand beginning to turn to hard skin, welcome. Join me in the glory of the latter years of life, the time when one should be able to enjoy retirement in peace and tranquillity, but beware the 'athlete passing the tape syndrome'!

At the end of the marathon the athlete passes the finish line and collapses. Yes, it's true he is obviously physically exhausted, but it's mentally that he has let go more than physically. Let's imagine that, without him being aware, we place the finishing line 10 metres further on. He would manage the last 10 metres without a problem. The letting go at the perceived finish is much more psychological than physical.

## WHEN TO RETIRE

A few years ago a retrospective study was done on two groups of people on reaching retirement. The first group retired at 60, and the second at 65. Both groups were followed until all the members of the groups had died.

Those who retired at 60 were shown to have an average life expectancy of another 17 years nine months. Those who retired at 65 had an average life expectancy of just an additional 18 months! Yes that's right, I didn't believe that either when I first read it. It's only when one explains the reasons that it all makes sense.

Let's take a look at the retiring at 60 group first, and to why they survived to an average age of 77 years nine months. At 60 they all felt young enough, and excited enough, to want to do something else. They felt physically capable of taking on a myriad of different tasks. Playing more golf, decorating the bedroom, planting that new rose bed. They didn't feel physically compromised by the passage of the years, and felt capable of taking on more or less any physical task. They were excited at the prospect of retirement as the beginning of a new dimension to life. Psychologically it wasn't the end of the marathon, but more the beginning of a new event. Psychologically it was an adrenaline-stimulating time.

Now let's look at the '65' group. We all begin to slow down a little as the years go by. Just as the first 20 years of life were a time of rapid change to our maturity, so too the last 20 or so are a time of decline. Energy levels that drove us to rise up the ladder in our working life begin to ebb. It becomes increasingly difficult to sustain the same pace that we managed so comfortably in our forties or fifties. Younger bucks in the herd are pushing from below to take our place. They threaten our composure with their energy. We are physically less capable and psychologically drained. We begin to mentally tick off the days until we can take that longed-for respite promised by the vision of retirement, and a rest from the physical and mental stress of our seemingly intolerable work life. We anticipate its arrival, and with that we lose the psychological drive necessary to sustain ourselves.

There's a good example of this from someone I met in my old running days. I can remember seeing his plight played out in front of the cameras of the world, as he staggered uncontrollably round the stadium at the end of the 1954 Commonwealth Games in Vancouver. Jim Peters entered the stadium at the end of 26 miles 385 yards of the Commonwealth marathon, or at least just one lap of the track left to complete the distance. The haven of the finishing line, when he was feeling so tired, was too much for his exhausted frame. The adrenaline spent, he pitifully staggered in total lack of coordination, from one side of the track to the other. Had that been another 300 yards along the road it would have been fine, it was the realisation that the finish was near that psychologically stopped the adrenaline drive, and led to the disaster. It was a terrible sight to see. Beware of entering the stadium of life's marathon; a similar fate may await.

## LAST OF THE SUMMER WINE

The quality of your latter years is really going to depend on how well you took care of yourself in earlier life. Has the wine matured well with ageing or has it been badly looked after and is now past its best? There is no doubt that the enjoyment of what should be the golden years in retirement can be sullied by our habits earlier on.

Many is the time a patient presenting with a persistently stiff and painful shoulder will say 'Why should I get this – I have played tennis all my life.' The thinking of 'use it or lose it' is fine to a degree. The other theory is, if you have a family saloon car and you tune it up to rally-drive every weekend, it's great when you are competing but not so hot when later you just want to use the car for shopping and leisure. It is bound to cough and splutter.

However, even if you have 'rally-driven' your machine almost to the breaker's yard, fortunately there is still hope. The body's powers of recovery are extraordinary.

## TOO MANY FLAT TYRES

Once over 65, and usually a lot younger, most of us will show the signs of having stood upright and of having sat for too long. Our children, now in their middle years, seem to appear taller. Of course they have remained the same; it is we who have shrunk a bit. It is our discs, between each vertebra, with the unsympathetic description of 'disc degenerative disease' that are the problem. The accumulated effects of lifting, carrying, standing and sitting have gradually squeezed the fluid from the discs and have left us with a series of flat tyres. The discs make up about a quarter of the length of the spine, so it doesn't take many 'flats' before the spine becomes shorter by an inch or so.

Postural habit, when we curved a bit too much from our dedication to the desk, adds to the appearance. Gravity, constantly compressing us to the ground, makes the curves a little worse and contributes to the loss of height. Don't worry too much about appearance – be it internal or external – it is how it works that is most important.

## STALACTITES AND STALAGMITES

We all at some stage in our education have seen photographs of caves where spikes of limestone grow towards each other. Remembering, I am sure, that 'tights come down, therefore mights come up', helps to remember that stalactites come down and therefore stalacmites come up. Centuries of dripping water in a cave allowed the formation of limestone deposits to build into the typical spikes that eventually join together. A similar process, gradually through life, works to our advantage by helping to stabilise our unstable discs. Let me explain.

When we damaged our discs earlier in life, we had recurrent episodes of back pain because the disc could wobble too much, which led to the reactive muscle spasm and chaos. Let's look at one over-wobbly disc, sandwiched between two vertebrae. All the time that disc, with its bulging 'tyre wall', is being compressed by

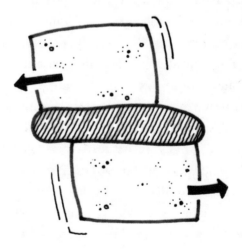

standing and sitting. The tyre wall, where it is attached around the rim of the bone, tries to pull away from its attachment. In a sense it tries to drag the edge of the bone with it. When you break a bone it is the tearing of the skin of the bone (the periosteum) that starts the process of new bone formation, to heal the break.

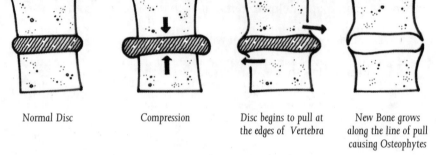

| Normal Disc | Compression | Disc begins to pull at the edges of Vertebra | New Bone grows along the line of pull causing Osteophytes |

**The Formation of Osteophytes**

To return to our wobbly disc; each little pull, where the edge of the disc is attached to the skin of the bone, drags the skin away from the underlying bone. As it does so, new bone forms along the line of the pull. All day, every day, the squashing of your 'flat tyre' gradually causes bone to grow around the edge of the tyre wall. On x-ray you can see these stalactites and stalagmites forming. They are your body's natural defence to stabilise your over-wobbly disc. Eventually these bony stalactites – osteophytes – meet and completely fuse, thus helping to stabilise the segment. Many times patients ask, 'Will I get worse as I get older?' The answer is 'no'. Most of the time your body will naturally help you.

There is a downside to all this. Unfortunately, some of these bony lumps can press on either the nerves, or actually into the spinal canal, and then cause problems that may require surgery to remedy. The principal thing is that as your back stiffens with the passing of years, it also becomes more stable, and so it is less likely to lead to those terrible bouts of acute chaos. Above all, don't fear a bad back. Use it regularly but with the wisdom of your years.

## KNEES, HIPS AND JOINTS

Joint problems are another product of standing on two legs. Standing on two legs has meant that the hips and knees have taken all the load of our weight-bearing over the years. Coupled with that, when our ancestors walked on natural surfaces, they didn't endure the unyielding concrete that we encounter every day. Soft ground absorbs the shock of our weight landing on one leg and then the other as we walk. With unyielding concrete the shock waves bounce back up, to be absorbed by knee and hip joints.

### Fair wear and tear

If I could, I would ban the word 'arthritis'. It is, at best, wrongly used and, at worst, too emotive. How many times has an insensitive GP or consultant given the patient the diagnosis 'arthritis'. The very word strikes fear and apprehension into most minds, conjuring up visions of a dismal future condemned to a lifetime of pain and suffering. The reality in most cases simply means a bit of wear and tear, the inevitable results of using structures for too many years. It is not necessarily the slippery slope to infirmity.

### The silicon-coated frying pan

When you bought that wonderful new frying pan, with its glistening grey-black surface, how well it cooked the eggs. No need for butter or oil; it was a perfect glistening non-stick surface that the eggs glided over. A few months down the line, a couple of scratches here and there on the surface, and you might need just a tiny bit of oil to stop the fried eggs from sticking. A bit more careless abuse and a bit of bare metal is starting to show through the now thinning silicon. Before you know it, it's either a resurfacing or a new pan needed. Take that metaphor and transfer it to a joint and you can now understand how joints work and how they wear out.

### The silicon-coated joint

Have you ever seen the blue-white glistening surface of a chicken knuckle? Or the round hip joint on a leg of lamb? Well, that's our silicon coating. It's not actually bone, it's articular cartilage. Think of it as being like the silicon on the frying pan, just as silicon is different from the metal underneath, so the articular cartilage is different from the bone underneath.

### Cartilage wear and tear

All the injuries – sudden and acute from jumping off a wall, or slow and accumulative from walking on hard ground – build up into wear and tear. Early on in our life we constantly renew the cells that form our bodies. New cells replace old; thus we keep resurfacing our joints. If the rate of injury outpaces the speed of renewal, or as the years go by, we don't repair as well and the articular surface begins to break down, we start to get the degenerative changes of wear and tear.

Our joints have a capsule enclosing them. The inner lining of the capsule is called 'synovial membrane'. Think of it as an oil-making membrane. Synovial membrane makes synovial fluid, which is your body's natural oil production unit. It keeps your joints oiled and the surfaces of your articular cartilage from getting damaged.

Now in this closed unit, microscopic-sized bits of the surface – of the articular cartilage – start to rub off. The minute particles of cartilage have nowhere to go and begin to irritate the synovial membrane, which does the only thing it can do – make more synovial fluid.

More synovial fluid is your body's natural solution to putting a bit more oil on the scratched silicon frying pan. Unlike the frying pan, which is only used once in a while, your hips and knees barely ever get a rest. They are always supporting you. As they continue to daily demand more oil to stop the surfaces sticking, gradually the overworked synovial membrane starts to thicken and get tired of the job. This is when you might notice that the knee is looking a bit thick and swollen. It also feels stiff after sitting for a while, or first thing in the morning. It's as if you have to 'get it going' before it functions normally.

What is happening is the production machine of your synovial membrane stops working at rest and needs the movement of your joints to 'milk' the production. First thing in the morning the joint is stiff, as the thick particle-laden fluid sticks across the joint, and prevents movement. After a few tentative steps, it begins to ease, as the movement increases the production of oil. Carry on too long and the production line cannot cope with the demand and it starts to get stiff and painful again.

Your doctor may initially prescribe some anti-inflammatory tablets. These will help to reduce the soreness of the overworked and inflamed synovial membrane, and early on in this story they can work wonders. You may also be sent for an x-ray.

Bone shows on x-ray because it has calcium in it. Cartilage doesn't show on x-ray because it doesn't contain calcium. So in a normal x-ray there is an apparent gap between the two bones. The gap is the depth of the articular surface – your 'silicon' covering. The amount of wear there is shown by how close together the two bones are. The closer together they are, the more you have worn away your silicon articular surface. Eventually, if it's not treated, you start to expose bare bone – you have got down to the bare metal of the frying pan.

## KNEE AND HIP REPLACEMENT

They seem to be two a penny these days. Hip replacement is becoming commonplace, closely pursued by the knee replacement. Some joints, both hip and knee, can be candidates for an interim measure – a resurfacing of the joint. This process merely replaces the articular cartilage, like having your frying pan resurfaced. Because some of your articular surface has not worn away and, as it is non-weight-bearing, areas of the joint can be salvaged. A piece of your own articular cartilage, about 1cm square in size, can be taken and grown in laboratory conditions until there is enough to resurface the damaged areas. This can only be done in the comparatively early stages of wear and tear, but for the right case it can be very effective.

### Total joint replacement

This means replacing the ends of the two bones and literally inserting a new metal joint. This operation has transformed so many people's active lives, and in the majority of cases is a great success. Ironically, the most worrying aspect currently is not the success of the operation itself but avoiding contracting a 'hospital infection' such as a 'superbug'. It will be interesting to see if the incidence of degenerative hip or knee disease diminishes in the future, when the generation who has worn trainers, with their shock-absorbing capabilities, rather than the leather-soled shoes of the current-65s and over, reaches the natural age for joint replacement.

Several years ago, a study was made of people showing evidence of the beginnings of the loss of articular cartilage (hip degenerative change), that involved getting them to wear shock-absorbing heel-pads in their shoes. If was found that there was a significant reduction in pain and stiffness and the deterioration rate slowed down.

We may find that trainers will protect the modern generation from the current high incidence of joint degenerative disease. I remember my mother aged 84 proudly buying her first pair of trainers. This helped her to cope with a painful bruised heel. So, whatever age you are, soft shoes will help you cope with wear in the spine and legs.

## Glucosamine Sulphate and chondroitin

Before closing this section, let me mention Glucosamine Sulphate and chondroitin. This is a food supplement that may help with the laying down of new articular cartilage. I mentioned earlier that in our youth – and, to a certain extent, in the middle years – we continually replenish our structures. Old cells die and new cells replace them.

Fortunately we are living longer, but this has its drawbacks in that we start to come into the age when our cells no longer replace themselves with new, and we simply wear out. For many, including myself, Glucosamine Sulphate and chondroitin seems to slow down that process and may even reverse it a little. It is worth trying a course. You can buy it at any chemist or health food store. Try it for three months. If you feel that the condition has improved, carry on. If there is no change, then stop. It definitely helps me. If I get out of the habit of taking it for a few weeks, I begin to notice that going up and down stairs becomes less comfortable. I start taking it again and I can almost run up the stairs!

## TAKING THE PAIN OUT OF GARDENING

There seem to be more problems in the latter years caused by gardening than any single other activity. Certainly, gardening is not only one of the best exercise therapies available but it also provides a mental discipline and interest. It's how you go about it that is so often the cause of back pain. You have to remember that 40 years, or so, of sitting married to the office desk has not naturally kept your musculature in the sort of state that can deal with a full day bending over a flower bed and digging. You will be fine if you keep taking frequent breaks; it's better to do short spells of different activities than one long session bending over weeding the garden path. So, do a bit of weeding, a bit of pruning, a bit of digging, and keep ringing the changes. You must behave like the athlete training for a marathon. Build up the ability of the body to cope with the new activity gradually. That way you will constructively gain fitness for the new tasks, and, more importantly, feel better for it.

### Fisherman's stool

Rather than bending over in the garden for hours, risking damage to your back, try sitting on one of those metal-framed folding canvas seats that you can easily carry around. Obviously, it won't work when using a fork or spade, so in that case, don't push your limits too far. It is much better to work for a series of short spells with a break in between, rather than attempt one long overtiring spell.

### Never kneel or squat

Knees are not only one of the most complicated joints but also one of the most weight-bearing. As we get older our ligaments, which join one bone to the other, become less resilient and this is the time to protect them.

Kneeling, with your lower legs on the ground and your backside on your heels, bottom resting on your calves, or just squatting on your haunches, puts an unacceptable strain on your knees. Get into the habit of avoiding this. When the knee is in one of those positions the musculature controlling the knee cannot come into play. The ligaments are bearing all the strain and, after 65 years of wear, are not capable of withstanding that sort of insult. If you want knees that will last a bit longer, then use the fisherman's stool and sit, rather than kneel or squat.

### Walk, walk, walk

Walking, preferably in trainers, is the best friend you can have to keep your body balanced and in tune. Remember that the aim is to keep good movement, to keep a comfortable rhythm, not to put you under unnecessary stress.

## SELF-ASSESSMENT

It's time to make a critical, one step away, look at the credits and the debits. Let's assume that you have just retired and want to enjoy those years of retirement to the full. Inevitably, some bits will have worn a little – some more than others, some less. It would be nice to identify those bits that need immediate attention and those that perhaps can be left alone for a while. Now that the pressures of the office routine, with the inevitable time schedule demands that this imposed upon you, no longer apply, this is the time to enjoy your freedom and make the most of your machine. To achieve the most success, you need, however, to exercise discipline. Now that you have the time available, use it wisely to protect the good bits and bring the slightly dodgy ones up to scratch.

Our National Health Service, I always thought, seemed more concerned with disease than health. However, current thinking, and action, is now more inclined to include health checks as a matter of routine. So take advantage of this new thinking. Go along to your GP and let him or her check out your medical fitness. Assuming that you receive no advice to the contrary, indulge in a little physical fitness programme. Not too much too quickly, but just enough to enable you to continue to improve daily. The rewards will be enormous.

In a medical sense, probably the most important checks are of blood pressure and cholesterol levels. These are the two factors that are universally accepted to contribute most to coronary disease, the biggest killer in our society, and that with sensible medication high levels can be substantially reduced. It's no use trying to get musculo-skeletal fitness if your arteries are clogged with the accumulated animal fats of dietary excess, and a high blood pressure that is trying to burst a hole in your ageing pipework. If you never managed to find the time to look at, and institute, some healthy eating regime, this is certainly the moment to do so. Don't just rely on the prescribed 'statins' and 'beta-blockers' from the pharmacy; start instead to take some responsibility for your own wellbeing. As with previous conditions, the more knowledge you have, the more you can make rational decisions for your present and future.

## WWW.STRESS

### What is it?
Stress merely describes the body's response to some form of external stimulus, be it physical or emotional. Without some level of stimulus we are barely able to function at all; it's the response mechanisms of how our bodies deal with stress that is so important to our survival.

### Why is it?
There are few people who have not heard of the classic 'fight and flight' response to a stressful stimulus. The flooding of adrenaline into the bloodstream and the subsequent release of the stressor, cortisol, is the body's reaction to a moment of fear that prepares it for action.

Unfortunately, with our modern sedentary life, often the only response available is merely to watch a screen or write an email – not the 'action man' response that nature has chemically prepared us for. The physiological changes in the body of increased blood pressure, higher pulse rate, channelling of blood supply to the muscular system and the fine-tuned, fast-acting nerve supply are fine for running down the jungle path, one step ahead of the pursuing sabre-toothed tiger, but are somewhat wasted if you just sit there clicking the mouse. The result is that without the 'action man' fight or flight response, cortisol builds up in the bloodstream and tissues and becomes an enemy, not an ally. The problem is that this state of alertness, triggered many times a day, has become a drug that the body is addicted to. When that suddenly stops at retirement age, this produces withdrawal symptoms. The body misses its 'adrenaline high' and this often leads to symptoms of anxiety and depression.

## What can you do about it?

The body was prepared for action and action is what it needs. Now that time is available, it can be well used in deliberate exercise. Some of the muscular pains, in the lower back and into the neck and shoulders, will certainly have been caused by the build-up of stressors in the muscle fibres. Similarly, the tense, hardened musculature across the shoulders and up into the neck and base of the skull is where the lactic acid will have built up as a result of insufficient natural movement to disperse it. Now is the perfect time to start exercising, if you have had years of inactivity. Your machine, probably rather neglected in the past, now needs your attention so that it can support and carry you through the enjoyment of your retirement.

Follow the simple stretching and exercising routines on page 206 to gently and efficiently restore movement, balance and strength to your precious machine. It's the only one you've got so it's worth a little effort to look after it. Regard it with pride, while you watch it improve with your efforts. If you have been prescribed beta-blockers, or some other medication to reduce blood pressure, then see if, by your own efforts to become healthier and fitter, you can get to a stage where, with your doctor's approval, you can either stop taking the medication completely, or at least reduce the dosage. That would be a tangible sign that your efforts are showing a really positive result. Take pleasure in this period of your life and celebrate the fact that, so far, you're a survivor.

## WWW. ANIMAL FATS

### What is it?

It's very simply the fats we ingest from eating meat and dairy products that have a high fat content and that contribute to coronary disease by increasing levels of cholesterol in the bloodstream.

Another disadvantage of a high intake of animal fats is that there is also a tendency to put on weight. The more weight you carry the more load you place on the joints, particularly the lower back and lower limbs. The adding of a few extra pounds is a constant burden to these structures, and something that with power and discipline can be changed.

### Why is it?

In our relatively affluent society, we have become used to ingesting increasingly high levels of dairy products on a regular basis. We happily pour the full-fat cream over our apple crumble, even though the pastry has been made with a hefty load of animal fat. Our urban environment, and with it the supermarket, has for years encouraged us to buy convenience foods such as high-fat sausages and bacon. Although many low-fat alternatives are now available, we find it relatively hard to buck this trend and make sensible dietary decisions for ourselves. A collusion of market forces is in part responsible for our high levels of cholesterol, and a contributory factor to our 'death by diet' coronary disease.

## What can you do about it?

Perhaps the best advice I can give you is to tell you a story about an area in Finland that in the 1970s had the highest death rate for coronary disease in the world.

North Karelia is, I understand, a rather cold and inhospitable region, lying close to the Russian border, and was the scene of a remarkable campaign that successfully changed the eating habits, and health, of its inhabitants. Before and during the Second World War, North Karelia was a typical area of Finland where the diet was simple and healthy; the main cause of death was from infectious diseases. The war over, and with a degree of peace and affluence entering the economy, eating habits began to change. With more available income, dairy products and sausages became the order of the day. A campaign was launched to educate and persuade the inhabitants to eat a diet containing less saturated animal fat and to instead eat more fruit and vegetables.

It was an impressive exercise in public awareness of a problem and it meant targeting both individuals and food producers to make it work. But work it did and the results were staggering. During the 25 years, between 1972 and 1997, when the project finished, deaths from coronary heart disease dropped by 82 per cent, cholesterol levels were reduced by 20 per cent and life expectancy in men rose by eight years, from 65 to 73!

Now that's something worth buying into if all it entails is a little self-discipline. With those figures in mind, why don't you sit down and take stock of what you buy and what's in the fridge. There are things to cut out, and there are things to add.

## Cut out

- Full fat milk, cream and butter.
- Fatty bacon, pork sausages and meat pies heavy in fat.
- Pies and pastries with a high fat content.
- Animal fat cooking oil.
- Dairy milk chocolate.

## Put in

- Skimmed or half-fat milk; vegetable oil spread.
- Lean meat, with the fat cut off if necessary; mushroom or vegetarian sausages.
- Fish, fresh or smoked.
- Vegetable cooking oils, such as olive or sunflower oil.
- Wholemeal bread with a low salt content.
- Plain dark chocolate (in moderation).
- Fresh fruit and vegetables.

I am sure that some of you will feel horrified at the thought of not having fatty sausages, bacon and pork pies. They are so convenient to eat and cook. But you will be amazed that, if you start not to have high fat foods in the fridge, how easy it becomes to get into good healthy eating habits. The potential reward of a longer healthier life may not seem so important in youth and middle age, but is inclined to focus the mind a little more in the later years when coronary heart disease strikes. So think about it. Of course it is your decision, but armed with this information, the effort might just seem worthwhile. You might even enjoy it!

## THE TEN-MINUTE DOZEN EXERCISE PROGRAMME

There are three essentials that we need for our musculo-skeletal health: mobility, muscular strength and coordination or balance. This programme will give you a mixture of all three elements and the opportunity continually to improve on your fitness levels.

### 1. Above shoulder arm stretches

■ Stand comfortably, with legs apart. Now, with palms facing in, reach up above your shoulders, trying to reach as high as you can with your hands. Then with alternate left and right hands try to reach for the sky. You should feel the inside of your upper arms brush your ears as you do it. Do 10 with each arm.

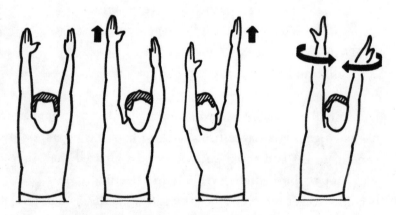

Exercise 1: Above Shoulder Arm Stretches

■ Next, with hands still held as high as possible, rotate the arms so that the backs of the hands face each other, then back to palms facing. Repeat 10 times.

■ Now let the arms drop down to your sides, and shrug your shoulders 10 times, making sure they rise as high as possible and then drop as far as possible.

■ Finally, relax and shrug your shoulders up and down a few times.

## 2. Trunk stretches and rotation

■ With fingers interlocked, place your hands on top of your head and then bend to each side in turn. Really feel your ribcage stretch as you bend to each side. Do 10 to each side.

■ Keeping your hands on your head, now try to slowly rotate your trunk to each side so that you look over each shoulder, behind you. Do 10 to each side.

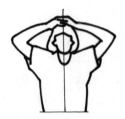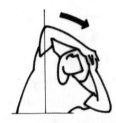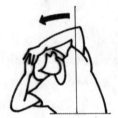

Trunk Side-bending

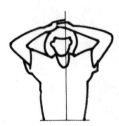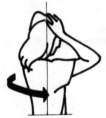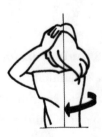

Trunk Turns

Exercise 2

## 3. Neck flexion stretches

■ Standing comfortably with legs apart, let your neck drop
   forward with the weight of your head stretching the back of
   your neck.

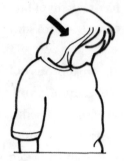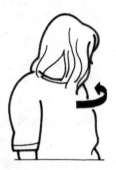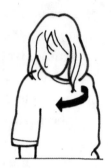

Exercise 3: Neck Flexion Stretches

■ Now rotate the head from side to side and feel the whole neck
   taking part in the movement. Always feel the weight of the
   head opening the back of the neck. Do 10 to each side.

■ Keeping your head hanging forward, now let your neck drop
   to each side, and try to touch your shoulder with the ear. Do
   10 to each side.

■ Now relax and shrug your shoulders up and down a few
   times.

## 4. Shoulder blades meeting at the back

This is familiar by now, I hope.

■ Stand comfortably, hands behind your back, and try to pull
   your shoulder blades back as far as they will go and at the
   same time feel the front of the chest opening up. Hold for five
   seconds. Repeat 10 times.

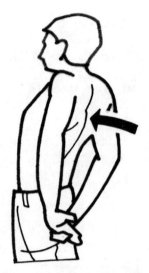

Exercise 4: Lumbar Extension

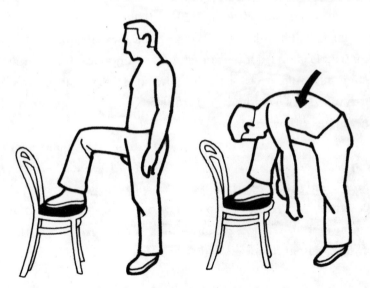

Exercise 5: Lower Back and Hip Stretch

■ Now relax and shrug your shoulders up and down a few
   times.

**5. Lower back and hip stretch** (see previous page for
illustration)

■ Put one foot up on a chair, or the side of the bath, depending
   on your chosen exercise venue. Try to bend forward to touch
   your toes and feel the stretch in your lower back and the hip
   and thigh of the raised leg. Do 10 on one side, then change

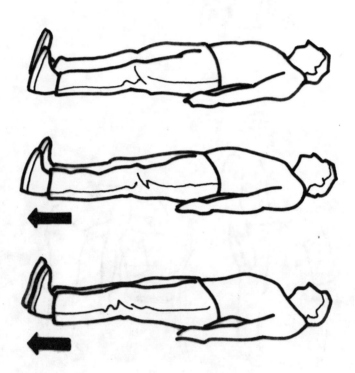

Exercise 6: Hip and Sacrum Slides

legs and repeat.

**6. Hip and sacrum slides** (see previous page for illustrations)
Lie flat on your back with your legs out straight and feet flexed to stretch the back of the thighs and calves. Now try to push alternate legs away, in the same manner as reaching above the head with your arms. You should be aware of your pelvis moving from side to side, and your sacrum being

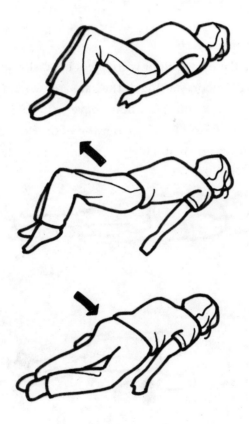

Exercise 7: Hip and Pelvis Rolls

manipulated between the two sides of your pelvis. Do 10 on each side.

**7. Hip and pelvis rolls** (see previous page for illustration)
Still lying on your back, bend your knees, with feet flat on the floor and then, with knees and feet together, let the weight of the legs roll you to each side. Try to keep the spine and trunk still and let the movement come from the base of the spine and pelvis. Do 10 to each side.

**8. Erector spinae lifts**
■ Still lying flat on the floor with knees bent, slowly curl your spine off the floor, starting at the base and working through one vertebra at a time. You don't have to lift high – just feel the spine begin to lift away from the floor. Hold the lift for five seconds and then slowly roll down and relax for five

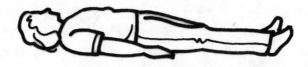

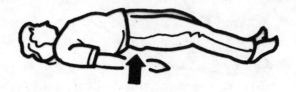

Exercise 8: Erector Spinae Lifts

seconds. Repeat. If this is too hard to begin with, just do as many repetitions as is comfortable, and gradually build up to 10 repetitions.

### 9. Abdominal curls

- Lie flat on the floor, with knees bent and feet flat on the floor, place your hands behind your neck and lift your head and shoulders off the floor. Hold for five seconds, then slowly return to the floor and rest for five seconds. See how many you can do comfortably and build up gradually to the full 10

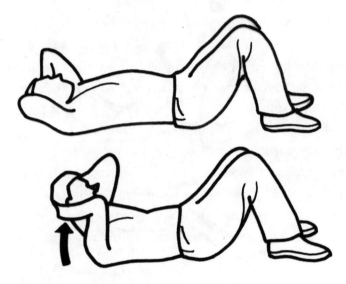

Exercise 9: Abdominal Curls

repetitions.

- When you can manage 10 repetitions comfortably, you can add a twist to each side so that the shoulder reaches towards the opposite knee. Build up to 10 repetitions to each side.

## 10. Dog stretch

This is our old friend from each morning. Remember, start on your hands and knees, arms straight and a little bit in front of the shoulders. Now drop your upper body forward, over your shoulders, allowing your back to curve fully into extension.

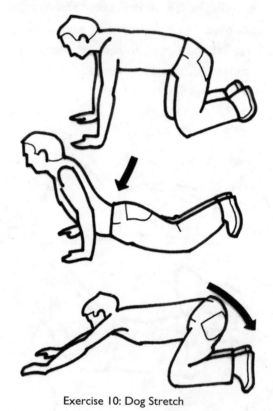

Exercise 10: Dog Stretch

Then, still with straight arms, lift your bottom and try to pivot back to sit on your heels. Accentuate the ends of each movement by holding in the position for a few seconds to feel the stretch all along the spine. Do 10 complete cycles.

## 11. Running on the spot

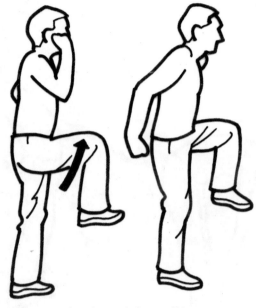

(*Raise knees as high as possible*)

**Exercise 11: Running on the Spot**

■ Try to lift alternate knees as high as you can as you run on the spot so that you feel your pulse rate going up. Try to keep going for one minute. See how many 'knees fully up' you can count in one minute.

## 12. Deep breathing

■ First shake yourself out a little. Shrug your shoulders up and down a few times and then let your arms relax by your sides shaking the arms and hands to feel them relax.

■ Now breathe in while raising your arms above your head to fully open the lungs. Then, when you feel the need to breathe out, bend forward and let the arms hang in front of you to try

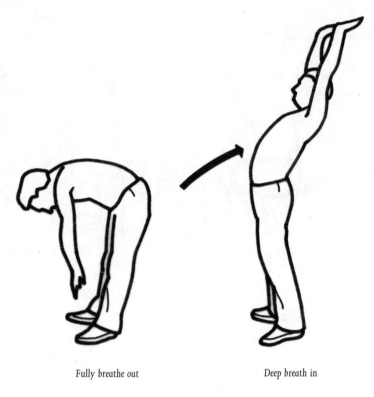

Fully breathe out                    Deep breath in

**Exercise 12: Deep Breathing**

and touch your toes. Only go as far as feels comfortable, but let the air empty out of your chest, holding for as long as possible until you feel the absolute necessity to breathe in again. You should aim to breathe out for longer than you breathe in. Slowly roll up again, and repeat. Start with just five repetitions, and gradually build up to 10. Also increase the length of time you hold the breath in and how long you breathe out and hold the position. This can be quite heady to begin with so only do it in your own time and capability. It's much better to build up gradually than to struggle too hard.

## HOW TO PROGRESS

Take a mental note of how far you were able to stretch and how many repetitions of each exercise you managed comfortably. Try to gradually improve on your score each day or every week.

When you feel ready, I would like you to build in an extra challenge in the first four exercises, where you are standing upright, and that's balancing on one leg! You may not be able to do this straight away but it is an aim for the long term. Wait until this routine is in your hard disc memory bank, and you do not have to think what comes next, before adding this variation. Start first by trying to stand on tiptoe on both feet. Once you are comfortable with this, then try to take more weight on one leg than the other while still keeping both feet in contact with the ground. Perhaps do five repetitions on one side and then five on the other. Progress to balancing fully on one leg, alternating the legs every five repetitions. Then you can move on to the ultimate challenge by balancing on one leg on tiptoe!

This is a complete body workout with the essential element of erector spinae – core muscle – balance and strength. The 'ten-minute dozen' will be a very good start to the day. If you really get the taste for exercise, there's nothing to stop you doing this several times a day if you wish. Don't forget also to walk, walk, and walk. Brisk walking is an excellent form of exercise and it's free.

# 14 BEDS, CHAIRS AND CHANGING THE ENVIRONMENT

The immediate environment is the one we inhabit for most of the day and every day, namely beds and chairs. We can comfortably cope with standing, providing we either keep moving or engage 'muscle control mode'; it's sitting and lying that present our biggest problem.

## SITTING AND LYING

Sitting and lying have one thing in common; they both involve ligamentous function. As I mentioned earlier, it's the ligaments that control our joint structures at rest. That's the time when we're not in muscular control of our 'performing seal on stilts'. If beds and chairs cause you to adopt a position that puts a strain on a ligament, at one end of its range of movement or the other, then it will start to hurt.

The simplest example of this is probably the ache you feel in the back of the knee if you rest one foot on a stool, with your leg straight, while sitting. With the leg unsupported, the back of the knee bends backwards into what is called hyperextension, and puts a stretch on the back of the knee. Spend a few minutes in this position and the knee will start to ache. To stop it you'll have to change position to take away the stretch on those aching ligaments.

The major requirement from both beds and chairs is to provide a comfortable neutral position for the spine. The limbs can cope, but the spine, with its multitude of joints, all with ligaments joining one vertebra to the next, needs sensible continued support. As soon as a segment, or a series of segments, is forced to the end of its range of movement unsupported, it will start to hurt. It won't stop hurting until the strain is taken off.

With that basic principle in mind, let's first have a look at beds.

## BEDS

Beds, or something to lie on, came long before chairs. The need to lie down for sleep has been with us for millions of years, while chairs have only been around for a few thousand years at best. I am sure that our early ancestors, though unaware of the concept of ligamentous function, must have sought a more comfortable resting place by lying on animal pelts, to soften the hardness of the cave floor.

Our ancestors' natural activities will have given them strong muscles with a higher resting tone, and since their lifespan was less than ours, they didn't survive long enough to develop degenerative diseases. Bearing that in mind, they probably slept pretty comfortably and well anyway. They would certainly not have suffered from staying with friends for the weekend, sleeping in the spare bedroom with its inevitable sagging old mattress!

Our problem is that we have become too weak to cope with a bad bed, be it too hard or, more likely, too soft. A choice of bed must always be in some ways be dependent on the person, or persons. Things to consider are how heavy you are and how you sleep. It's not only your weight but perhaps your partner's as well. Many are the times that I have heard that the expensive new bed suits one partner but not the other. Do you sleep on your front, back, side. Do you toss and turn around a lot, or do you stay very still? The bottom line is that the bed must be neither too hard nor too soft. The ideal bed must at least allow you to wake without back pain.

My first, and really only question, when asked to comment about a patient's current bed is, 'Do you wake up feeling worse in the morning than when you went to bed?' If 'yes' then a follow-up is, 'Have you slept in any other bed recently where you were able to wake pain free?' If that is the case, you must find out the make and category of that bed. Make a careful note of it and keep it for when the time comes for you to buy a new one.

Beds may sometimes seem to be a rather expensive item. Yet if you look at the cost against the amount of time that it's used, then the price of even the most expensive of beds can seem to be good value. Let's say that roughly a third of your life is spent in bed. Allowing time for being away from home, let's round that down to 300 days in bed per year. Again rounding down to eight hours per night we are looking at about 2,400 hours per year. Take the lifespan of a good bed to be at least ten years then that would be 8000 hours of use. Even if you spent £1000 on the bed, which is at the upper end of the range, it amounts to only around 4p an hour! Not bad value for a good night's sleep.

For any bed to be any good it must fill a few criteria. Too soft will be as much, or more, of a disaster than too hard. The ideal bed needs a top surface that enables you to sink into it a little so that your curves may be accommodated. If the top surface is too hard, then, if you were to lie on your side, your hips and shoulders would be supported, but not your waist. In that case your spine would be forced to curve down towards the bed's surface to gain support. This will place a strain on the ligaments so that if the pain doesn't wake you, it will certainly cause problems in the morning, and getting out of bed will feel like a major effort. The combination of your weak ligaments, from being too sedentary, and some disc degeneration cause the vertebrae to sink out of line. This means you are effectively having to stack them one on top of each other to straighten up.

If you're lucky, gradually standing upright permits the muscles to gain control and with a bit of walking, in muscle mode, you can re-establish your authority over your aching spine. However, if you're unlucky, a bad bed can trigger a full-blown flare-up of any old back problem you may have had. It could even be the trigger for a weakened disc to finally blow and cause a 'Full Monty' sciatica, ending up needing a neuro-surgical operation.

The moral of the story is get a good bed and don't stint on it. It's cheap in the long run! However, I always advise against getting an 'orthopaedic' quality bed as these are usually too hard. They seem to have evolved from the idea that 'if a hard bed is good, then a harder bed is even better' principle, which isn't actually right. Many patients have given me very good reports on Tempura mattresses. They are designed to sink with your weight and then support you.

The best thing is to go to a reputable store, one that carries a good selection of beds, and to ask the salesman for his view and advice. There are always so many new variations being

developed, that it's only those working at the cutting edge who
know what is available. To recap, too hard a bed will be as much
a disaster as too soft. Think of a soft-top surface that can support
you comfortably and then the rest of the mattress should be firm
enough to stop you sinking too far.


## CHAIRS

Apes don't sit on logs. But we do . . . Then we made them into
desks and chairs and really screwed up!

Sitting is one of the most unnatural activities that we perform.
And if sitting is bad, then chairs are even worse – we certainly sit
on them for far too long. The basic problem is that sitting is a
static function and chairs are inert.

Let me explain a little further. When we are on the go it's a
dynamic activity that involves movement and muscular function
to control it. We deal with that pretty well, as it's very much the
activity that we have in common with all other animals on this
planet. Sitting, on the other hand, is a non-muscular activity that
engages ligaments which can't be actively controlled like
muscles. This means that we don't manage sitting very well, and
unfortunately our modern world demands that, one way or
another, we have to spend a large part of our waking, and
working, life doing it.

It's only in the last 20 years or so we have really started to look
at the design of chairs to be functional and not just pretty. The
act of sitting in a chair is an inactive function and, even worse,
it's performed under the vertical compression of gravity putting
inevitable pressure on our long-suffering lumbar discs. The net
result of that is an ongoing disaster. Yet, with a little thought,

based on the understanding of the problems involved, then chairs could be designed to be a lot more user-friendly. We also need to sit in them correctly. That means sitting right back in the chair to ensure the correct support is available. The trouble is that having, at some considerable expense, bought the top-of-the-range model, most people then just sit at the front of the chair, leaning over a desk to work at their computer. For all the good that it's doing them they might just have well bought a wooden bench!

When we sit at the front of a chair we inevitably slump our weight with our lower backs curved out to the limit of flexion (forward bending). In this position our unsupported weight compresses the discs in the base of the spine and at the same time forces the ligaments to be stretched to their limits. Remember that ligaments are the straps on the 'Mini' door, and that if you lean against them they will gradually stretch and inevitably get longer. The longer, and therefore more lax, the ligaments become, the less they are able to stabilise the joints that they control.

The chair that I favour, and use, to sit at my desk and sometimes when treating a patient, is the 'kneeling chair'. I am absolutely lost without it, though many people think they look awful. The trouble is that we have become so indoctrinated to look at a chair in a particular way. We need a radical rethink about chairs if we are to survive comfortably in our modern sedentary world. We need to get away from 'designer' concepts and look at it instead as a design exercise in function. We need a chair that interacts with us in such a way as to demand muscular control that will, in turn, protect our ligaments.

Certainly I suggest you try one of the kneeling chairs available on the market. It will take a few days to get used to it, but once you have tried it you'll almost certainly be hooked. The major principle is that we need to maintain the natural inner curve at the base of the spine. That's what the kneeling chair very effectively achieves. At the same time, because it rocks slightly, it demands gentle muscular balance from you – back to the old story of proprioception – your body's balance awareness in space. It thus fulfils the two criteria of maintaining neutral posture and encouraging active muscular control.

## MAKING THE MOST OF WHAT YOU'VE GOT

Adapting any existing chair can work by just putting a cushion in the small of the back.

People love to slump in their favourite armchair or sofa in what they think is a comfortable position. The reality is that, after a few minutes, they are fidgeting around to find another position that will relieve their ligamentous discomfort. Throw away your preconceived ideas of comfort in a soft sofa and instead try a more upright chair with a cushion in the small of your back. You'll find it much more comfortable in the long run. The same advice applies for when you're in the car.

Remember, sitting is very unnatural, so try to make it as natural as possible by maintaining the inherent curves of your spine. As always, knowledge is your strength. It enables you to make rational decisions for your own wellbeing. Ultimately it's your body and it's your responsibility. All I can do is give you the information and point you in the right direction – the rest is up to you.

# 15 OSTEOPATHY, CHIROPRACTIC AND PHYSIOTHERAPY

'What is the difference between osteopathy, chiropractic and physiotherapy?' This is a question that I must have been asked thousands of times over the years, and yet it is one that I still find difficult to answer adequately. Searching for a simple yet accurate description while being bombarded by news reports of the latest political party conference season gave me an idea.

The differences between osteopathy, chiropractic and physiotherapy are in many ways similar to the differences in Britain's current political parties. Each major party – Conservative, Labour and the Liberal Democrats – is offering to manage the country, and cure its ills, by slightly different methods. The country remains the same body of structure and function, yet each party feels that its special approach and philosophy will work best. That is exactly the way in which the three disciplines of osteopathy, chiropractic and physiotherapy are operating and thinking. We are all dealing with the same body – its structure and function remain the same; it's only our approaches to its management that are different.

Let me give you a little background to the three disciplines, their origins and beliefs. Fortunately I have good credentials to talk about all three, as i have been an osteopath for more than 40 years, had a father who was a chiropractor for 65 years and I am still involved in the teaching of post-graduate courses in osteopathy for physiotherapists.

## OSTEOPATHY

I will start with osteopathy, as that has been the label under which I have plied my trade. American physician Andrew Taylor Still is credited with founding osteopathy in 1874. As a practising doctor in the Midwest of America he became disillusioned with the ability, and resources available, to satisfactorily treat disease. In this environment, one that lacked the medical knowledge and treatments of today, Still proposed his simple, but revolutionary theory, that the body is a self-contained, self-healing unit, and that with a suitable understanding of the body mechanisms of physiological repair one could learn to both speed up this process, or free up any obstacle preventing its perfect function.

Embraced within this concept were two pillars of wisdom that supported these views: 'the rule of the artery is supreme' and 'structure governs function'. 'The rule of the artery is supreme' simply means that a healthy blood supply, and good venous and lymphatic drainage, is likely to support a healthy environment. That's what I outlined at the beginning of this book, when I talked about the loss of drainage mechanism that occurs when using a computer mouse, and how this can lead to repetitive strain injury.

I can think of no finer example of 'structure governs function' than my earlier description of how the elevation of the first rib prevents the normal elevation of the shoulder in a rotator cuff lesion (see chapter 6). Remember the student who had been unable to elevate her arm beyond the horizontal for 18 years. The dramatic change that occurred when I corrected the problem in the first rib is a testament to this concept.

With these two principles Still had a practical basis on which to found a new profession and establish a school to teach its message. My only argument with this is that he chose to call this new profession osteopathy! This has led to the mistaken belief that 'osteopaths treat bones'. We don't really treat bones in fact we may treat everything else in the body, be it muscle, ligament, tendon, fascia or organ, but we merely use bones as levers to work on those structures.

In the limited medical environment that existed at the end of the nineteenth century the osteopathic doctor flourished and reputations grew. 'The rule of the artery is supreme' and 'structure governs function', Still's two principles, were put to practical use, for example, in treating a case of pneumonia – a potentially serious infection of the lung. The osteopathic physician would attend frequently at the patient's bedside and work to increase the motion of the ribcage and unblock any relevant dysfunction of the vertebral column, to not only improve the blood supply but also increase venous and lymphatic drainage, the osteopathic physician's recipe for health. It is not difficult to imagine that, given the medical treatment of the time – sulphur drugs, blood letting and purging – the osteopathic patients had a more sporting chance of survival by enabling the body's own medicine chest, within the immune system, to play its evolutionary and vital role in maintaining health.

In today's medical climate, few patients or practitioners would opt for osteopathic treatment, given the proven efficiency of antibiotics in such circumstances. There may come a time, however, when our profligate use of antibiotics, and the resultant resistant strains of bacteria, renders our current antibiotics obsolete. We may then have to resort to working with the body's vast store chest of naturally occurring remedies, available in the bloodstream, to effect natural resolution to infections.

Still's osteopathy and his school in Kirksville, Missouri, grew and flourished. As the twentieth century unfolded, so osteopathy expanded and more schools opened – all teaching a natural concept of medicine founded on his basic rules. Two figures emerged, both graduates of the school at Kirksville and students of Still, who were to become especially influential in the development of osteopathy: William Garner Sutherland and Martin Littlejohn.

Sutherland's influence, through intelligent thought and observation, was to detail the motion, and importance, of the cranial bones and the effect they have on body function, known as the cranial mechanism. His truly pioneering work is still carried on today, with thousands of osteopaths around the world able to provide non-invasive treatments for a myriad of problems from glue ear to giddiness, and sinusitis to sciatica, as a result of his teaching.

Dr Martin Littlejohn's unique contribution was to found the British School of Osteopathy in 1917. His inclination was towards physiology – function rather than structure – and contributed much to the physiological understanding of our profession.

In Britain in the 1930s there was an abortive attempt to establish osteopathy, via a parliamentary act, as a legally constituted profession that would have been acceptable in the same way as the then newly established dental profession. Until then, dentistry and osteopathy could be practised by anyone with just the desire to do so. No official qualification was necessary, you could, if you wished, just put up a plate saying 'Dentist' or 'Osteopath' and open the door to any willing patient.

The failure to gain full parliamentary recognition for osteopathy left the profession in a somewhat bruised state and lacking self-confidence. In this tentative condition, we seemed to lose sight of the potential that osteopathy can offer, and were prepared instead to settle for being some sort of super physiotherapy, highly skilled in manipulation, limited to only treating musculoskeletal problems. Because the common public image of an osteopath is of someone who treats 'bad backs', it tends to ignore many of the functional medical problems in which osteopaths may also excel. Fortunately at the end of the 1960s, the Sutherland Cranial Teaching Foundation started a programme of lectures that was to change osteopathic thinking and reinstall a belief in the treatment of functional problems.

Let me give you an example. A patient whom I had known for many years happened to mention that his six-year-old son had received six courses of antibiotics, over the last year, for a recurrent sore throat. When I suggested he bring him in to see my colleague, my patient justifiably asked, 'What does your colleague do?'

'He's an osteopath,' I replied. 'What on earth has an osteopath got to do with sore throats?' was the inevitable response.

My colleague, a contemporary of mine from the British School of Osteopathy, has for some 30 years specialised in treating children, and ranks as one of the top few in the world of paediatric osteopathy. I explained to my patient that if after several attempts to treat his son's throat problem with antibiotics there was no real improvement, there may be some factor preventing the normal function of the throat. My patient was not totally convinced but agreed to see my colleague. Three weeks later, when he came to see me again, he was bubbling over with enthusiasm and said, 'After the first treatment my son was much better, and now after two more sessions he is totally clear of sore throats and is a different child. He just seems to have so much more energy.'

My colleague, Stuart Korth, and I discussed the problem and apparently the child had a very restricted upper ribcage that was preventing normal venous and lymphatic drainage, effectively causing a 'damming up' of fluid drainage from the throat. Simply releasing this restriction not only cured the throat problem but also improved his breathing and his overall vitality. Another clear example of the 'structure governs function' principle.

The collective anecdotes of colleagues across Europe would fill many volumes, and I'm sure inspire much support from grateful patients, as stories like these abound. I doubt whether any osteopath, currently in practice, would consider osteopathy to be an alternative system of medicine, capable of competing on equal terms with current medical practice, as it did in Still's time, but rather as having a complementary role. As conventional medicine seems to be becoming more and more removed from the patient, relying on a battery of tests and computer read-outs that define your ills, patients are disillusioned by rarely seeing the same doctor twice. They crave some sympathy, and a bedside manner that treats them as a human being and not a series of statistical possibilities. It is in this field that osteopathy can flourish and make a real contribution to health in a practical and realistic manner.

## CHIROPRACTIC

Chiropractic and osteopathy share enormous common ground and yet have many differences. I hope that I won't offend chiropractors by not giving as deep a history and background as I have for osteopathy, but my personal experience of chiropractic is obviously not as great as that of my own profession.

During his teens my father was treated by a chiropractor for severe asthma. Asthma, a condition affecting aspects of breathing, may be regarded as a functional condition in that there is usually no demonstrable pathological cause. He must have been very fortunate, in that he was treated by one of the first chiropractors in the UK.

It has been said that chiropractic came as an offshoot from osteopathy. It was founded by Daniel David Palmer, who focused on spinal manipulation as a treatment. One of the differences was that chiropractors believed any vertebral misalignment caused bony pressure on nerves, leading to problems not just in the surrounding muscles and tissues but also in other areas of the body. The osteopathic concept was more that any physiological changes in a disturbed spinal segment would affect the surrounding autonomic nerves and lead to an impaired blood supply to any tissues supplied from that level. These differing concepts led to a difference in approach. Chiropractors tend to focus much more on direct manipulation to the spine with short sharp thrusts, or adjustments, while osteopaths, though using manipulation, tend to take a more subtle approach, often using the bones as levers to change the surrounding soft tissue structures. In essence chiropractors are more concerned with the relative position of a vertebra and osteopaths more with the motion of the segment. This is reflected in the pattern of a treatment session. Frequently a chiropractic treatment can be 10 or 15 minutes in length and consist of just specific manipulation, that is a short sharp thrust resulting in an audible crack. Some chiropractors, though by no means all, often insist on patients having a course of 36 treatments, three a week, then two, then one and then to have regular maintenance once a month. I find this in direct contrast to the fine osteopathic maxim, 'Find it, fix it and leave it alone'.

I think it is fair to say that osteopathy takes a broader approach, as it embraces many different methods of treatment other than manipulation. However, I understand that some chiropractors are now embracing some of the principles of cranial motion. Both professions, especially when it comes to treating musculo-skeletal conditions, will be addressing the same structures and be using predominately manipulative techniques. In truth, there are so many variations between individual practitioners of both disciplines, and how they apply their treatments, that from the patient's perception there would seem to be no hard and fast rules. The most obvious difference they might encounter would be a cranial osteopath who didn't use manipulation and a forcefully adjusting chiropractor who did nothing else.

## PHYSIOTHERAPY

Physiotherapy is the odd one out in the trio. It does not have a specific philosophy of approach but instead is a medical auxiliary profession. Not so long ago, physiotherapists could only treat a patient with a referral from a GP or a consultant who made the diagnosis. It was then for the physiotherapist to carry out the prescribed treatment accordingly. They were the 'physical arm' of medical therapy for rehabilitation and remedial exercises. Now physiotherapists have to take a four-year degree course and have a far greater autonomy in deciding the nature of the problem and the treatment necessary. Though patients can elect to see a physiotherapist, it's still more common for them to be referred by a medical practitioner.

Physiotherapists are at their best in organising and supervising exercise programmes for rehabilitation of anything from a stroke to a sprained ankle. They also tend to use various electrical therapies such as short-wave diathermy, ultrasound or heat lamps as part of their therapy. As with most professions there is an immense difference between the 'very good' and the 'not so good'. The 'very good' are highly responsible practitioners, capable of taking decisions over the treatment of their patients, and offering swift and sure recoveries from a variety of physical conditions. I am afraid that the 'not so good' can be found in some hospital physiotherapy outpatients departments switching on and off heat lamps, with the patient getting better in spite of the treatment rather than because of it.

## THE OVERVIEW

Osteopathy and chiropractic both have philosophies that separate them from the conventional medical approach, whereas physiotherapy is a part of the Health Service. Osteopathy and chiropractic perhaps share the most similarities, although osteopathy has a broader canvas on which it operates, and tends to use more gentle methods of treatment. However, all three professions are statutory self-regulating bodies and have contributions to make to the nation's health, and all help in reducing absenteeism from work through back pain.

# 16 A FEW EXPLANATIONS

## X-RAYS, CAT SCANS AND MRI SCANS

The wavelength involved in x-rays is so penetrating that it can break down the bonds that bind chemical structures together. The code present in every cell in your body, the human genome, is made from the chemical substances called nucleotides – notes that build up into long chains of DNA melodies that are the instructions to build the proteins of which you are made.

The ionising radiation in x-rays can potentially disrupt these connections and therefore disrupt the code, and can in some cases trigger cancerous changes in the body. You only need one wrong note, in a chain of several thousand, to change the code and trigger a possible cancerous change in the body.

Fortunately, repair mechanisms are constantly at work to keep your code intact. It's only when some factor prevents the repair that disaster may unfold. The ionising radiation that was released into the environment several years ago with the Chernobyl disaster caused massive changes in the DNA instructions and led to large-scale outbreaks of cancers. We have polluted our world with various sources of ionising radiation that is described as at acceptable background levels. Like a mathematical equation, adding A B and C together may add up to more than an acceptable level, though A B or C may individually be described as acceptable.

We undergo a constant check on our DNA links – the chemical bonds that link long chains of amino acids – and we are constantly repairing the damage to the sequences of nucleotides that code the building of normal healthy cells. Failure to carry out quick and efficient repair may result in cancerous changes. Recent investigation has shown that low-level radiation, as with x-ray, may postpone repair for several days, whereas a higher level of radiation stimulates a speedier response. So sometimes a low level dose of radiation can be potentially more harmful than a high one. The simple answer is to be aware of risk and take responsibility for your own wellbeing, it's too late after the event.

GPs and consultants are frequently guilty of demanding pictures, when a good case history and a brief physical examination would have revealed just as much, if not more. Remember, three x-rays a year is thought of as the upper limit, and one-third of that is unnecessary unless there is a massive and good reason for doing so. Don't be pushed into it; we have enough background radiation without adding unnecessarily to the risk.

It seems there is a greater fear for the medical profession that not having x-rays and scans may pose a risk of medico-legal action, should some case be made against them for professional negligence. The potential, always present in our economically minded society, of litigation can often outweigh good case history based clinical judgement.

I find it particularly prevalent in the field of musculo-skeletal medicine where x-rays very rarely contribute much to the treatment and diagnosis of the problem. The patient is never really given much option in the decision, though. My advice is to ask if x-ays are essential and if your doctor or consultant

convinces you of the need, then go ahead, but let him know that
you need to be informed of the risks.

## CAT SCAN

CAT stands for Computer-Aided Tomography. By taking a series
of x-rays at various levels of focus a picture is built up which, with
the aid of a computer, can show a 'slice' through you. In lay
terms, it would be better to call it computer-aided 'slice'ography.

Think of a machine in the supermarket slicing ham. To begin
with, all you can see is the outside of the ham block. As the
machine cuts you your six slices, and they fall slice by slice onto
the waiting paper, each slice is a 'tome'. You can look at each
tome and see the amount of fat, the blood vessels cut across – the
whole interior is revealed.

A CAT scan simply takes a series of slices through you with a
very controlled x-ray-based camera, so that sections of you can be
recorded on the negative of an x-ray plate or looked at directly on
a computer screen. The computer software then enables the
images to be enhanced, enlarged or viewed from different
directions. Direct the slice to the right level and it can reveal, for
example, a bulging disc pressing on to a nerve root leading to
perhaps the excruciating pain of sciatica.

A word of caution. Ingenious as it is, this is not a procedure
without hazard. A lot of x-ray radiation is necessary to take all
these pictures, so don't be subjected to this onslaught unless there
is a major gain to be had from it. You are always perfectly justified
in asking for an explanation as to the nature of the procedure,
what it entails, what are the risks and what is the potential gain.
Your consultant may be a bit put out by your questions but do

satisfy yourself that you are quite happy with what's being done to you.

## MRI SCANS

MRI stands for Magnet Resonance Imaging. It shares the same slicing principle as a CAT scan but replaces the potentially dangerous x-ray with a very powerful electromagnetic field. Everything – you, this book you are reading, the chair you are sitting on, the air you are breathing – is made up of atoms. Electrons spin around a central nucleus in each atom. By imposing, very briefly, a massive electromagnetic force – sufficient to arrest the spin of each electron – and then record its return to normal on stopping the field, a picture is built up. Every tissue – every bone, nerve, blood vessel, tendon and ligament – has a special resonance that can be read in this manner. The negative, like an x-ray plate, gives the best detail yet available of our inside. It can help to show our structures, hitherto unseen. The cautionary note here is that the electromagnetic field is enormous and may not be totally harmless. It is too early to tell yet, but err on the side of caution.

## CRANIAL OSTEOPATHY

In this country cranial osteopathy is a new concept and treatment. It has its origins through the persistent curiosity of an osteopathic student, William Garner Sutherland, eventually coming to fruition as a treatment method in the mid-thirties.

William was a pupil of the founder of osteopathy, Andrew Taylor Still, at the original Osteopathic Medical School at

Kirksville, Missouri. History has it that students were encouraged by Still to look at the skeleton and critically analyse its function, and that Sutherland was almost obsessed by the way the bones of the skull fitted together at the sutures, in such an intricate yet ordered way. Following the osteopathic philosophy that structure governs function, he spent his life's work trying to understand what was the function of the skull bones, with their facility for motion, other than forming the bony box for the brain. It was his studies that led to the understanding of the role of cranial motion in health and disease.

I touched on this topic in chapter 13. However, I would like to give you my personal view of what is cranial osteopathy and its significance as a method of treatment. I must say that, like many of my contemporaries who have been educated in a very structural concept of osteopathy, the idea of these apparently palpable subtle motions having real effect was rather inconceivable. I hasten to say now I would be at a great loss if I did not use cranial techniques and palpation.

In order to explain we need to go back to birth, or really to conception. So come with me on a little journey that I fully accept is largely hypothesis, and certainly most of it very difficult to prove.

At that extraordinary moment of conception, when two living cells coalesce, and share their genetically coded information, begins a new individual. At that moment is written a code, that will organise and construct a new human being, grow it to maturity, and run it for the rest of its life, maintaining it in health and providing methods for its healing.

The basis of osteopathic medicine is that the body is a self-healing unit, and that the osteopath, by understanding body function, is there to assist that process, or unblock any factor that may be preventing the body's ability to restore itself to health. Sometime after conception it is said that the embryo begins a motion that will remain for the rest of life. This consists of a rhythmic lengthening and narrowing, followed by a shortening and broadening. A rhythm that is repeated, from the beginning of one phase to the start of the next, at about a 10-second cycle. This is entirely involuntary; hence the more accepted title of 'involuntary mechanism', rather than cranial osteopathy. It varies from person to person, and can show marked variations under different circumstances.

So what is it?

I don't think anyone really knows, but those who use it have their own ideas and I would like to give you mine as I have no doubts that it has significance in the quality of our existence.

If one thinks of the intelligence that was present at the moment of conception, and that that intelligence has been able to organise the building of a complete human being, in some five or six months, then there has to be some intelligent organisation to control and monitor this. As the embryo is making these extraordinarily complex and rapid changes in growth there has to be some feedback to check that everything is in order, in the right place and functioning. This cranial motion acts like a radar beam, expanding and contracting, like the tide on the shore, reporting back, as it were, the state of every cell that integrates to form us. In a sense it is the interface between the structures that have been built and the intelligence that has built them.

In a practical sense when one 'tunes in' to this involuntary mechanism, you pick up an awareness of not only the part that you are in contact with at the time, but a sense also of the whole body, relative to that part. You can feel whether the part you are holding is in unison with the whole, or seeming to be out of phase with it. Holding the particular unit, allowing it to balance in your hand, you can the allow it to join in unison with the rest.

I can only give you an example that happened to me when I took my first 'cranial course' some 30 years ago at a post-graduate conference in Belgium. For several months prior to the course I had suffered from a left-sided acute sinusitis. I had been treated by a colleague, swallowed medication, inhaled steam, and had all sorts of treatments, conventional and alternative. All to no avail. At the end of the first day of the course we had finished the programme rather earlier than anticipated, and the American osteopath leading the team suggested that, rather than leave early, we might take the chance for one or two of us to be treated for something. We were three students to a treatment table, with one professor per table. I leapt in before anyone else at our table could get a look in and asked if Herb Miller, our teacher, would look at my sinus problem. I lay on my back on the plinth and he felt over my maxillary sinuses and said that the zygoma – the bone under the orbit of the eye – on my left side was blocked, and not allowing for the drainage mechanism to function properly. With a barely perceptible touch, he placed his index finger over the zygoma. He seemed to rest it there for a few minutes and then said, 'I think that should allow it to work a little better now.' I thanked him, but secretly thought what a complete load of rubbish.

Walking back to the hotel that evening, I discussed this 'non treatment' and dismissed it as a waste of time and money to have come here if that was all that it was about. I woke the next morning and was rather surprised to realise that I had slept without pain, and couldn't even seem to remember which side was the painful one. I have never had a moment of problem with that sinus to this day. I must tell you that I did thank Herb Miller for not only the treatment but also for the very practical lesson.

Cranial osteopathy is a difficult one to understand until you have experienced it yourself.

# 17 A LAST WORD

## THE PAST

Time now for a moment to reflect on our journey from the past, our time in the present and a thought or two for the future. We have come a long way since our ancestors left behind those telltale footprints in the volcanic ash at Laetoli. We will probably never know what they looked like, how they communicated and what were their thoughts about the world they lived in. Yet these are the things that preoccupy us so much in our literature today. Sadly, without time travel or the benefit of art left behind, these insights must remain tantalising mysteries.

I think it is safe to speculate that our ancestors probably didn't suffer the same sorts of back pain that have come to dominate our current existence. For sure they had back pain, but probably from injury and not indolence. Without doubt their lifespans were shorter and therefore they suffered fewer of the age-related degenerative conditions. I doubt whether there was the same prevalence of disc injury, as the innate muscular support of active, daily used, erector spinae muscles would have ably supported the spine and protected the discs from compressive forces. Those early bipedal relatives were so fresh from the trees that they must have been lithe and musculo-skeletally fit. Their only real concern was survival in the harsh school of nature.

What on earth would they make of their offspring if we could suddenly confront each other and show them what a journey they began for us, and where we have taken it. Which brings me to the present.


## THE PRESENT

We do need to improve our present lot; we can't tolerate the levels of back pain and absenteeism from work that currently prevail. The problem is essentially the same one as in North Karelia, where, as relative affluence prevails, we indulge ourselves to the extent that we start to behave in ways that lead to our downfall. The heart disease that developed from our self-indulgent and lazy eating habits is no different from the musculo-skeletal dysfunctions that have come about because we have lost our natural 'diet' of athleticism. We are in physical terms, at the interface of our own evolution. Our sedentary 'diet' is the cause of our progressive sliding into increased back pain as we fail – with increasing incidence right from childhood – to use the muscular equipment that we possess. Use it or lose it, in our case, really does apply.


## THE FUTURE

Unless we either change our environment or ourselves, we are going to be the increasing victims of our evolutionary pathway. We have arrived at a situation where we seem to be at a bottleneck. Our structural evolution, far from going forwards seems to be on the decline. The evolution, meanwhile, of our intellect is producing an increasingly sedentary existence, not only for us but also more worryingly for our children. We may –

just as we find ourselves increasingly under surveillance with cameras at every street corner – find ourselves sliding inevitably into a combination of George Orwell's *1984* and Aldous Huxley's *Brave New World*.

It took a pioneering project, over 25 years, to change the lives of the Finnish population of North Karelia and to give them improved health and increased longevity. If you were to follow the suggestions outlined in this book, you could make a material change to your own life in 25 days!

There is no need to be the victim of back pain. All you need is to understand the reasons for it occurring and follow the simple steps I have given you to be the master of your own destiny. All that you need to do is to make a commitment to want to change, and then the rest is easy. In fact once you start it just gets easier, as you load into your body's hard drive the conditioned reflexes of habit. Bad habits are easy; the good ones need a little application.

There is a lovely saying that was told to me, and that you can repeat to yourself as a meditation mantra each morning. I have often given copies of it to my patients, who tell me they have it above their bathroom mirrors. It goes thus:

'This is the start of a new day. When this day ends I will have exchanged one day of my life for what takes place. Let it be for good not evil, for gain not loss, for happiness not sorrow, that I may truly say at the end of the day that the exchange was worthwhile.'

Those are somewhat philosophical thoughts, but let them take on a more tangible meaning by resolving to start each day with the will to be in charge of your own machine. Take pride in controlling your body, rather than being the ship that, without steering, becomes the victim of the prevailing elements and ends up on the rocks.

I have given you the knowledge and the tools to make realistic change. The only thing I cannot do is to do it for you – that's your responsibility.

# GLOSSARY

'The body doesn't call it the acromio-clavicular joint' wrote Rollin Becker, an American osteopath. In the English language, it is accepted that the small joint that joins the collarbone to the acromion process of the shoulder blade is named the 'acromio-clavicular' joint. It is of course very convenient, for anyone in a medical field, to have universally recognised words to precisely identify an anatomical structure. However, when we lift up the arm at the shoulder, and motion occurs at the AC joint, isolating that structure by naming it totally fails to give an insight into the complexity of how the body organises and synchronises itself to perform that task. It's a sad fact that naming things in this way often precludes an understanding of their function.

Rollin Becker's simple sentence had a profound effect on the way in which I try to visualise structures that I feel with my hands. It almost seems that attention to naming them limits the 'experience' of them.

That said, you may find it helpful to have a glossary of some of the words used in this book, and to divide the body into systems that share a common function.

## NEUROMUSCULOSKELETAL SYSTEM

This is without doubt the most important system in the body. Though we revere the specialists in the fields of cardiac, gastric, renal, liver and reproductive disease, all of these fields, and the systems they incorporate, are merely back-up facilities for the physical activity of the body.

We are active beings and action is all about the neuro-musculoskeletal system. It consists of: -

■  The central nervous system
■  Nerves
■  Muscles
■  Bones
■  Tendons
■  Ligaments
■  Fascia
■  Articular surface
■  Synovial fluid
■  Synovial membrane
■  Capsule
■  Intervertebral discs

## THE CENTRAL NERVOUS SYSTEM.

This is the hub of our action and control. It consists of the brain and spinal cord.

■  The brain

Our mainframe computer that organises and controls our every action and thought. On it we load the software programmes of our knowledge, be it the language we speak, the musical instrument we play or the golf swing we don't quite master. It is without doubt the most complex structure in our world.

■  The spinal cord

The main pathway to convey messages from the brain to the rest of the body be it to organs or the vital musculoskeletal structures that are the core of our function. Not only carrying action (motor) signals to the structures but also information (sensory) signals from the structures to the brain.

■ Nerves

These are divided into motor, sensory and autonomic nerves.

Motor Nerves carry signals from the brain to the muscle with a command for muscle fibres to contract.

Sensory nerves carry signals that enable us to 'sense' our body. Heat, cold, touch and orientation in space – proprioception – are the principal messages that are carried back to the brain.

Autonomic nerves deal with our household management systems. As the word implies, they are not under our conscious control, but take place automatically. They serve to balance our internal world against the world outside. They control, for example, the calibre of our arteries, constricting or dilating them to balance our temperature and blood pressure.

■ Muscles

The great bulk of our body that enables actions to take place. Each muscle consists of millions of microscopic fibres, which, under signals from the nervous system, can contract. The collective contraction of groups of these fibres, enables the acts of power and delicate control that are the feature of the muscular system and the very means of our everyday life.

■ Bones

Bones are the levers that muscles control to make movement of our bodies possible.

■ Tendons

Tendons are the 'ropes' that at one end are attached to bones and at the other to muscles. Muscles exert a pull on a tendon to move a bone at a joint.

■ Ligaments

Ligaments are the straps that join one bone to another at a joint. They are richly supplied with nerves and sensitive to stretch, so

that as fibres of a ligament start to be stretched nerves are stimulated to make the muscle contract to prevent the ligament being
strained. Too much force, or too quick an action, and you can
sprain or tear a ligament. The continuous stretch of a ligament in
a vertical posture provides the muscular stimulation for
maintaining balance. Ligaments and their nerve endings are the
instruments of proprioception – the sense of spatial awareness.

■ Fascia

Fascia is the prolific white connective tissue that envelops
everything in our bodies from organs to muscle and bone. It's like
cling film dividing and packaging muscles and organs into
compartments. It's the white under surface of skin – revealed with
a deep cut. It's everywhere and yet its absolute function is still not
well understood.

■ Articular surface

Articular surface or articular cartilage is the blue-white covering
of the ends of bone at a joint. It's the silicon surface of a frying
pan. It's the smooth, non-stick, friction-less bearing surface
that enables our joints to move so easily. Once it gets scratched,
just like the frying pan it is no longer perfectly non-stick and
begins to wear away. It needs to be constantly bathed in
synovial fluid.

■ Synovial Fluid

Synovial fluid is the joint oil that bathes the surface of the
articular cartilage and prevents wear. It is made and secreted by
the synovial membrane.

■ Synovial Membrane

Synovial membrane continually manufactures synovial fluid and
joint movement releases it into the joint. It is the inner lining of
the joint capsule.

■   Joint Capsule

The joint capsule contains the joint. It is attached from one bone to the next, completely sealing, enclosing and protecting the joint as a watertight unit.

■   Intervertebral Discs

The intervertebral discs are the specialised washers between each vertebra. They permit motion of the spine, and act as shock absorbers. They are made of a tough outer casing, the Annulus Fibrosus, and a gel-like core, the Nucleus Pulposus.

■   The Annulus Fibrosus is the tough outer casing of the disc that has to withstand the tons of compression that we daily subject it to when we lift vertically. A gradual weakening of part of the outer wall can allow a bulge to develop, and fluid from the core to seep out in the manner of a slow puncture in a car tyre. This loss of pressure in the disc – our tyre – leads to instability and allows one vertebra to wobble on the one below. If the process continues the weakened disc wall may permit a herniation, with pressure on a nerve sometimes leading to sciatica. A sudden force can cause the outer wall to burst leading to a ruptured disc.

■   The nucleus is the gel core that provides shock absorption and the distribution of load from one vertebra to the next. It is the essential component of our upright posture.

THE VASCULAR SYSTEM

If the neuromusculoskeletal system is our very being and function then it is the vascular system that is the 'life blood' that keeps it going.

It consists of:

■   The heart

- The blood vessels
- Blood
- Lymphatic system

## The Heart

The heart, the core of the system, distributes blood to the body by the rhythmic pumping of the muscular walls of its four chambers. It receives 'spent' blood from the body and pumps it through the lungs to absorb oxygen in exchange for carbon dioxide. The oxygenated blood is then returned to the heart to be pumped round the body to complete the cycle.

## The Blood Vessels

These are the arteries, veins and capillaries that form, with the heart as the pump, a continuous containing network for the distribution and return of blood to the body.

- Arteries are the muscular walled tubes that carry blood from the heart to every cell in the body. A build up of fats in the blood stream, in the form of cholesterol, can block the walls of arteries and impede blood flow. If this occurs to the arteries supplying blood to the heart muscle wall, it can result in a cardiac infarct – a heart attack – due to loss of essential oxygen to the tissues and the resultant death of the relevant muscle fibres.

- Veins are the non-muscled tubes that carry blood back to the heart. They have to rely on either gravity, or the contraction of muscles, to assist their function. Sitting for too long without movement, as in a long plane journey, can prevent the flow of blood, particularly in the calf muscles of the lower leg, allowing the blood to clot in the veins leading to a deep vein thrombosis. On later movement the clot may break away from the wall of the vein and move along the veins to the heart or lung to cause an embolism. This may lead to death through lack of oxygen supply.

■ Capillaries are the small, sometimes microscopic, vessels that are the final distribution channels to all the tissues of the body. They are very delicate and are susceptible to damage from pressure, with blood then leaking out into the surrounding tissues and showing as a bruise or haematoma.

■ Blood Pressure. In order for the system to work it is necessary for a degree of force to permit the flow of oxygenated blood to every part of the network. Too much pressure will damage the tubes; too little will result in a failure to distribute the vital blood supply to where it is needed. Blood pressure is maintained by the action of the autonomic nervous system on the muscular walls of the arteries. Signals to contract the arterial walls will narrow the tubes, while relaxing the muscle wall will widen them. By constriction and dilation of different sections of the network blood supply can be varied according to need. Though blood pressure varies slightly from person to person, 120/80 is generally accepted as the normal figure. The two readings represent the heart contracting and dilating – systole and diastole. The lower figure is the pressure in the system between heart beats, the upper is the pressure induced in the system as the heart beats. The more constricted the arterial system the higher the blood pressure (hypertension).

■ Blood.

Blood is a colourless liquid that appears red due to the presence of red blood cells. It's a constantly changing substance that nourishes, protects and provides the energy for our function.

▓   Lymphatic System.

The lymphatic system is a remarkably diffuse system of ducts and tubes that drain lymph from the tissue spaces back to the heart and vascular system. Through a series of valves (lymph nodes) it acts as a filter system to protect the body from the spread of infection. Hence the swelling of lymph nodes in infection and in the spread of cancer. It is also a drainage mechanism through the skin, via a vast network of miniscule lymphatic ducts.

# INDEX

Figures in italics refer to
illustrations.